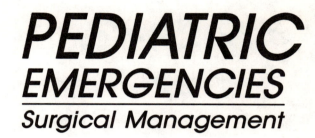

PEDIATRIC
EMERGENCIES
Surgical Management

PEDIATRIC EMERGENCIES

Surgical Management

JAMES C. FALLIS, M.D., FRCSC

Former Director, Emergency Medical Services
The Hospital for Sick Children
Toronto, Canada

B.C. Decker Inc.
Philadelphia • Hamilton

Publisher   **B.C. Decker Inc**
One James Street South
11th Floor
Hamilton, Ontario   L8P 4R5

B.C. Decker Inc
320 Walnut Street
Suite 400
Philadelphia, Pennsylvania   19106

Sales and Distribution

United States and Puerto Rico
Mosby-Year Book Inc.
11830 Westline Industrial Drive
Saint Louis, Missouri   63146

Canada
Mosby-Year Book Limited
5240 Finch Ave. E., Unit 1
Scarborough, Ontario   M1S 5A2

Australia
McGraw-Hill Book Company Australia Pty. Ltd.
4 Barcoo Street
Roseville East 2069
New South Wales, Australia

Brazil
Editora McGraw-Hill do Brasil, Ltda.
rua Tabapua, 1.105, Itaim-Bibi
Sao Paulo, S.P. Brasil

Colombia
Interamericana/McGraw-Hill de Colombia, S.A.
Carrera 17, No. 33-71 (Apartado
Postal, A.A. 6131)
Bogota, D.E., Colombia

Europe
McGraw-Hill Book Company GmbH
Lademannbogen 136
D-2000 Hamburg 63
West Germany

France
MEDSI/McGraw-Hill
6, avenue Daniel Lesueur
75007 Paris, France

Hong Kong and China
McGraw-Hill Book Company
Suite 618, Ocean Centre
5 Canton Road
Tsimshatsui, Kowloon
Hong Kong

India
Tata McGraw-Hill Publishing Company, Ltd.
12/4 Asaf Ali Road, 3rd Floor
New Delhi 110002, India

Indonesia
Mr. Wong Fin Fah
P.O. Box 122/JAT
Jakarta, 1300 Indonesia

Italy
McGraw-Hill Libri Italia, s.r.l.
Piazza Emilia, 5
I-20129 Milano MI
Italy

Japan
Igaku-Shoin Ltd.
Tokyo International P.O. Box 5063
1-28-36 Hongo, Bunkyo-ku,
Tokyo 113, Japan

Korea
Mr. Don-Gap Choi
C.P.O. Box 10583
Seoul, Korea

Malaysia
Mr. Lim Tao Slong
No. 8 Jalan SS 7/6B
Kelana Jaya
47301 Petaling Jaya
Selangor, Malaysia

Mexico
Interamericana/McGraw-Hill de Mexico, S.A. de C.V.
Cedro 512, Colonia Atlampa
(Apartado Postal 26370)
06450 Mexico, D.F., Mexico

New Zealand
McGraw-Hill Book Co. New Zealand Ltd.
5 Joval Place, Wiri
Manukau City, New Zealand

Portugal
Editora McGraw-Hill de Portugal, Ltda.
Rua Rosa Damasceno 11A-B
1900 Lisboa, Portugal

South Africa
Libriger Book Distributors
Warehouse Number 8
''Die Ou Looiery''
Tannery Road
Hamilton, Bloemfontein 9300

Singapore and Southeast Asia
McGraw-Hill Book Co.
21 Neythal Road
Jurong, Singapore 2262

Spain
McGraw-Hill/Interamericana de Espana, S.A.
Manuel Ferrero, 13
28020 Madrid, Spain

Taiwan
Mr. George Lim
P.O. Box 87-601
Taipei, Taiwan

Thailand
Mr. Vitit Lim
632/5 Phaholyothin Road
Sapan Kwai
Bangkok 10400
Thailand

United Kingdom, Middle East and Africa
McGraw-Hill Book Company (U.K.) Ltd.
Shoppenhangers Road
Maidenhead, Berkshire
SL6 2QL England

Venezuela
Editorial Interamerica de Venezuela, C.A.
2da. calle Bello Monte
Local G-2
Caracas, Venezuela

NOTICE

The authors and publisher have made every effort to ensure that the patient care recommended herein, including choice of drugs and drug dosages, is in accord with the accepted standards and practice at the time of publication. However, since research and regulation constantly change clinical standards, the reader is urged to check the product information sheet included in the package of each drug, which includes recommended doses, warnings, and contraindications. This is particularly important with new or infrequently used drugs.

Pediatric Emergencies: Surgical Management   ISBN 1-55664-298-9

Library of Congress catalog card number: 90-82201   10 9 8 7 6 5 4 3 2 1

Foreword

During the past 15 years tremendous strides have been made in the management of surgical emergencies. Much of this has come about because of vastly improved diagnostic techniques, especially in the field of radiology, but an even greater component is due to the training of physicians, especially primary care physicians, in emergency medicine and surgery. Most community hospitals are now staffed by such physicians, who do periodic shifts in the emergency department, and it is to these that Dr. Fallis' book is primarily addressed.

The book reflects Dr. Fallis' dedication to children and the experience he has gained through years of dealing with them and their parents as Chief of the Division of Paediatric Surgery in a large community general hospital and Director of Emergency Services at The Hospital for Sick Children, Toronto. His introduction should be *"must"* reading not only for physicians dealing with children in an emergency department, but also for all physicians dealing with children anywhere.

The tempo of illness in children is what sets them apart from their adult counterparts. They become ill quickly, and they may die quickly, but they have tremendous recuperative powers, and with proper diagnosis and treatment they recover quickly.

Dr. Fallis stresses the importance of history taking and a thorough physical examination. Although time-consuming, it is time well spent, and most diagnoses are made on this basis, with tests being mainly confirmatory. It is a time to establish rapport, to gain the respect and trust of both the child and parents, and will save countless hours in the long run. There is nothing more rewarding than the mutual trust and respect engendered by a good physician-patient-parent relationship, and as Dr. Fallis states "this is best obtained and maintained with kindness and a sense of humor."

Dr. Fallis stresses the importance of "inspection" (don't do something—stand there, and observe the child), learning to recognize a "sick" infant or child, and leaving uncomfortable hands-on maneuvers, such as palpation, until the end. In fact, abdominal examination and checking for tender areas or a stiff neck can often be carried out quite unobtrusively while talking to the parents and child.

The text is simply and beautifully presented, and it is difficult to single out particular areas of excellence and importance. The chapter on "Lacerations and Suturing," explaining how to do the job painlessly and how to deal with a moving target, is especially relevant to all emergency departments. The chapters on "Acute Abdominal Pain" and "Recurrent Abdominal Pain" deal thoroughly with perhaps the most common and potentially serious presenting complaint of children. The chapter on "Gynecologic Emergencies" by Jennifer Blake, M.D., is a very welcome addition to an often neglected area.

The book is liberally laced with pearls of wisdom gleaned from Dr. Fallis' broad experience—pearls such as "shock in a patient with a head injury," or relatively simple lacerations and trauma, often means an associated problem such as a ruptured spleen.

Although written particularly for the family practitioner working in the emergency departments of community hospitals, or the emergency physician in a mainly adult hospital where an occasional child appears, I would strongly recommend this book for pediatricians and for residents and interns dealing with children.

HARRY BAIN, M.D.
Professor Emeritus of Paediatrics
University of Toronto
former Physician-in-Chief
The Hospital for Sick Children, Toronto

Preface

It is my hope that this volume will assist in the management of infants and children with surgical conditions, both major and minor, seen in emergency departments or physicians' offices anywhere. If a result is that one child has less pain, fewer threatening tests, a quicker and more decisive diagnosis, it will all have been worthwhile. If this outcome is achieved many times for many children, it will have been worthwhile many times over.

In arranging the material, I have attempted to include information not readily available elsewhere. Indeed, I hope that what has evolved at least in part is a collection of "pearls" learned from a great many others as well as from the experience of 15 years in pediatric general surgical practice and 15 years with duties, both clinical and administrative, in a busy pediatric emergency department. This volume is far from encyclopedic. The obvious gaps in areas where there is no particular difference in the management of the child from that required by the adult are intentional. This is not a comprehensive text and should be used as an adjunct only.

As a pediatric general surgeon, I could be considered overly presumptuous for trespassing in foreign territory when I discuss topics normally taught by orthopaedic, plastic, ophthalmic, or neurologic surgeons or dentists. To the contrary! I feel the lack of a vast knowledge in any one of these areas is to a degree what permits me the effrontery of discussing them. The teaching of a subspecialist naturally reflects his or her subspecialization and generally presumes much in the way of background information. My lack of an extensive background knowledge in each of the specialties removes the risk of presuming it in my readers.

Indeed, I have the best of all worlds in that I have the privilege of writing on topics for which others stand as the acknowledged experts, while at the same time having the interest and total cooperation of those selfsame experts who have very generously reviewed the manuscript and provided their "oh so tactful" comments. I cannot describe how supportive and reassuring they have been, and I extend sincere appreciation to those who have given their time and effort in this way. They are listed under Acknowledgments.

I have long had association not only with primary contact physicians, but also with first-year family practice, emergency medicine, and pediatric residents, interns fresh from medical school, and student clerks. I hope this exposure has taught me how to present the material in a way which should be both readable and usable for those seeing children in the office or emergency department.

Some practitioners just naturally get along with children and need no advice on how to approach them. Others have absolutely no rapport with young patients, will never acquire it, and should spend their days dealing with dead tissue, test tubes, or adults. On the other hand, one frequently meets the individual who has not previously had the opportunity to deal with children, either in youth organizations or family, and needs a few pointers before trying to assess for the first time a totally uncooperative 4-year-old whose anxiety is matched only by his mother's. In the Introduction, I have tried to present some of the techniques which have worked for me in these difficult situations, although the reader will doubtless develop his or her own methods as time passes. While doing so, it must be remembered that "the young child is not just a little adult" (this is a cliché which all writings on dealing with children seem to incorporate). When confronted with a "difficult" child, the first thing to do before approaching too closely is to stop and think about how to obtain and maintain rapport.

The Introduction also contains information on some of the other general aspects of pediatric primary surgical care, although much of it is not unique to surgery, and concludes with a brief description of the principle which I have used for some time in trying to teach students and house staff how to avoid missing serious disease.

As in most emergency publications, the emphasis in this book is on diagnosis and initial care. For those not being admitted, I have tried to cover treatment from start to finish. For those with more serious conditions requiring admission, I have kept the discussion of treatment, for the most part, to the first hour or two in the department, although with a few conditions I have alluded to long-term care and prognosis.

Generally I have chosen to omit those conditions rarely if ever seen in the emergency department. Those conditions not generally considered to have surgical implications are discussed only insofar as differential diagnosis requires it.

The main focus of this book is the primary contact physician confronted by the ill or injured child who is as yet undiagnosed, not the consultant physician or surgeon who will bring to the patient the special knowledge which for the most part is omitted from these pages. Accordingly situations or conditions are described in which "referral" or "consultation" is given as the recommended management but in which many emergency physicians might be perfectly capable of continuing further. Indeed, there are countless hospitals in which the full spectrum of specialists is not immediately available and in which the emergency department staff must make decisions and initiate treatment measures considered in other institutions to be within the domain of the consultant. I ask that these competent emergency experts not take affront because in some areas I have elected not to go into the depth they might have preferred. I have tried to keep the material comprehensive rather than intensive in order to produce a final product of practical and useful size.

Acknowledgments

I owe sincere appreciation to my colleagues in the Division of Emergency Paediatrics at The Hospital for Sick Children for their encouragement and advice and to Dr. David Jaffé who succeeded me as the director of the division and of the Emergency Services. His support has been very important in the completion of this project.

Although the manuscript was recorded directly on a word processor, the many earlier editions and revisions of the booklet from which it evolved were typed and retyped countless times by my secretary, Mrs. Anna Capizzanno. Her efforts to maintain accuracy and a continuing high quality have been crucial in the ultimate product and are greatly appreciated. The line drawings were capably produced by Ms. Sari O'Sullivan.

Chapter 32, Gynecologic Emergencies, was written by Dr. Jennifer Blake, Gynecologist-in-Chief, The Hospital for Sick Children.

Consultants who have reviewed portions of the manuscript include Dr. John Wedge (Orthopaedics), Dr. Ronald Zuker (Plastic Surgery), Dr. Harold Hoffman (Neurosurgery), Dr. Raymond Buncic (Ophthalmology), Dr. David Wesson (Trauma Service), Dr. William Holland (Radiology), and Dr. Douglas Johnston (Dentistry).

JAMES C. FALLIS, M.D., FRCS(C)

The orientation talk given to every affiliating intern arriving in the department by Dr. Stuart A. Thomson during the 8 years he served as Surgical Supervisor was the stimulus for the production of this book in its initial form. After many revisions its purpose is still to perpetuate, in some small way, the teaching he provided.

Contents

Introduction

Assessment

The child in the emergency department because of a surgical condition may be totally cooperative and may pose no particular difficulty when the physician attempts to obtain a history and carry out an examination. On the other hand, the patient may be frightened or in pain or perhaps just spoiled, belligerent, and ill-behaved. In any of these instances, assessment can be very difficult, and all your patience and resourcefulness may be required. Remember two important things—*smile* and *go slowly.*

Although firm discipline is occasionally needed to handle a child, this is the exception. Generally rapport is best obtained and maintained with kindness and a sense of humor. Even though a child irritates beyond measure, *smile.* Let no evidence of irritation show. Do nothing that has an aura of ominousness or foreboding. Intimidation prevents communication.

Avoid startling or frightening a child with too quick an approach or sudden movements. Move slowly. Do not palpate until you have obtained a complete history, watching the child all the while. Inspect thoroughly before palpating. When touching, try to distract the child. If you can direct attention to something other than your examining hand, a reaction that seems to be in response to pain is more likely to be spontaneous and honest. Do not cause pain until it is necessary because doing so may remove all possibility of obtaining any further useful information. Do not tell a frightened child to move his or her arm: hand the child something and watch. Do not order a difficult patient to walk across the room: ask his or her mother to move away and watch the child get to her.

When you sense that a child is going to be difficult to examine, stop and ask yourself how you will best be able to obtain the needed information. Try to dream up the trick or subterfuge that reveals what you need to know without the child realizing he or she is being examined.

Assess to the best of your ability and recognize that the assessment may take much longer than it would were the patient a cooperative adult. Inadequate examination is caused more often by unwillingness to spend the needed time and effort than by lack of knowledge or experience.

Try to reach a working diagnosis before requesting any special investigation. The presence of a presumptive diagnosis on the radiograph or laboratory requisition implies that the child has been assessed carefully and completely.

Investigation

Laboratory tests and radiographs are important but are never justified unless they are likely to contribute to diagnosis or management.

A radiograph requisition is a request for a radiologic consultation. The medical information on it should include a brief history, relevant findings, and the physician's best attempt at a provisional or working diagnosis. The site of trauma should be recorded because this is not only essential to the radiographer who takes the x-ray films, but also to the radiologist who interprets them. Do not hesitate to discuss the case with the radiographer, who may have valuable suggestions about special views or the usefulness of the ones you have requested.

The degree of detail warranted for investigation in an emergency department is different from that appropriate for inpatients. For practical purposes, tests in the emergency department should relate only to the complaint with which the patient presented to the department and not to other conditions, pre-existing or unrelated, unless one suspects the presence of a serious or life-threatening illness. Strictly speaking, no more investigation should be done than is necessary in the decision to admit, to substantiate, or to rule out an emergency diagnosis or to facilitate emergency care. However, if unrelated symptoms suggest the presence of an additional condition that requires elective assessment, the emergency physician is obligated to communicate this to the patient's regular physician.

Subsequent venipuncture tests beyond those needed in the emergency department are sometimes ordered on a sample of blood from a child who is being admitted in the hope of avoiding the second venipuncture after the child reaches the ward. This is justified only if one can be sure that the tests actually are not repeated on the ward. More extensive investigation is also sometimes warranted when a child who does not require admission has come from far away and would otherwise need a second elective visit to complete a needed work-up. These considerations are all relative, however, and take low priority when the department is busy.

In spite of the frequency of situations that have legal implications, physicians must guard against requesting expensive investigation solely for legal indications. In such instances the quality of patient assessment and the careful recording of it is of far greater importance.

Treatment

For patients who require admission to the hospital it is important to make the appropriate referrals to the inpatient service as soon as possible. Initial investigation and treatment measures must be started at once. However, when a different medical team will be caring for the child on the ward, it is desirable for those physicians to be involved as soon as the transition can be made easily and smoothly.

Of those children who do not require admission, some need no specific treatment beyond reassurance. If this is the case, that should be the extent of the treatment. Do not treat just for the sake of doing something. If antibiotics are not indicated, do not order them just because a parent requests them. On the other hand, a patient's regular physician may have led the parent to expect admission, a certain procedure, or a specific medication, none of which may be felt by the emergency staff to be indicated. When this is the case, careful reassurance and complete explanation are required and must be done without criticism of the patient's regular physician. Ideally you should discuss your decision with the outside physician before instituting treatment, although practical issues frequently prevent this. At any rate, you should proceed with the proper treatment after explaining your decision to the parent.

If treatment once started in the emergency department needs to be carried on outside, be sure that all the necessary arrangements for this are completed.

Communication

When a child goes home from the emergency department, it is important that parents be told clearly what to expect and particularly what danger signs to watch for. On leaving parents should know what to do, whom to call, and where to go if the child's condition worsens or fails to improve as anticipated. This advice is very important— almost as important as the accuracy of diagnosis and appropriateness of treatment. It provides parents with something to fall back on before they see or can contact their own physician. The discharge advice and the telephone number of the emergency department, often printed on a tear-out sheet for parents, provides security, both medical and legal, that can be obtained by no other means. It is important to record on the chart exactly what the parents were told.

Be sure all follow-up arrangements, with family physicians, regular pediatrician, or clinic, are completed. Record on the chart what these arrangements are.

If you think you are not communicating satisfactorily with the parents, ask someone else to try. If language is a barrier, request an interpreter. Be sure that the interpreter explains all instructions carefully and tells the parents where to telephone or what to do if progress is not as expected.

Dealing with Parent and Child

Unfortunately child control is sometimes more like disaster control. The scenes in which it takes four people to control a screaming toddler so the physician can look in his or her ear or both parents and a frustrated nurse to restrain a child so he or she can have a hand sutured are certainly unacceptable and usually unnecessary. From time to time one must treat a retarded teenager who has no control over his or her reactions and may have the size and strength of an adult. However, these situations are very unusual. For the most part, even the hysterical child who needs surgical repair of a laceration, removal of a foreign body, or establishment of a venous infusion can be dealt with expeditiously, in a businesslike manner, with a minimum of commotion.

The value to a child of the presence of a comforting parent is well recognized, and current teaching recommends that parents be with a frightened child whenever possible. Fortunately most parents are able to remain controlled and calmly reassuring during procedures. Consequently, in most instances presence of a parent not only supports the child, but also can facilitate the procedure.

Unfortunately, this positive role is not true of all parents. Apart from the parental tendency to faint when everyone's attention is directed to the job at hand, some parents are emotionally incapable of the supporting role and can make the procedure very difficult. Sometimes a parent who may even realize that he or she should not go into the treatment room with the child will insist on attending because of the mistaken belief that it is a parental duty or obligation to be present as an advocate for the child, almost as a protector against "attackers." In this situation the young child may continue to cry and yell at the parent to "rescue" him or her as long as the parent is present. One wonders if the memory of being "tied up" and "mommy just watched and wouldn't rescue me" might be more damaging than the procedure itself. Crying toddlers stop crying sooner and more consistently when there is no parent to whom to cry. Surely the child who stops crying quickly and can then be engaged in conversation during the remainder of the procedure has a healthier recollection of it than the one who cries throughout, whether or not a parent is present.

Although parents' rights may include being in attendance during basic examination and treatment procedures, fortunately the majority do not insist and agree to leave when asked to do so. When they do, parents should be placed out of earshot and not left to stand listening outside the door. Indeed, when the procedure goes well and the child becomes calm and willing to converse with the staff, it can be very reassuring to anxious parents if they are summoned to see this for themselves at the end of the procedure.

Appropriate and effective restraints are a necessary "evil" in pediatric emergency departments, although it is perhaps better to run the risk of having to interrupt a procedure to apply restraints that were initially not thought to be needed than to apply them to a child who would have cooperated without them. Restraints may be more traumatic to the child than the procedure itself and should not be used unnecessarily. However, when applied to a small child for a procedure requiring him or her to keep still, struggles usually stop quite quickly when it is apparent that they are accomplishing nothing. Local restraints, such as one applied to a hand and forearm when a finger is being sutured, are also of great value and too often neglected.

The general image displayed by the physician in charge of a procedure is important in determining the response of the child and has a strong impact on the parents if they are present to see it. The physician is in charge, and it must be evident that this is so. If the child needs to adopt a certain position, or if something unexpected becomes necessary, this is done because the physician requests it and not because "mommy wants you to" and certainly not so the child can earn a promised reward after everything is finished.

The physician who is uncertain what to do next during a procedure is asking for failure of cooperation. Children tolerate badly those physicians who make unnecessary moves, who continually stop, and who waste time. One must try to use an economy of movement, to do what is necessary and no more, to be as expeditious as is consistent with doing the job well and, so far as is possible, painlessly.

For even the most irritating child, or the one who is the most difficult to control or restrain, the physician must still put maximum effort into examining or treating the child as skillfully and with as little discomfort as possible. A child's inability to cooperate at a tender age during a treatment procedure is no justification for less than optimum results which the patient will continue to live with for decades. In addition, when a laceration is sutured virtually painlessly but on a child who could do nothing but fight and cry throughout, there is one maneuver that may help the child to accept better the procedure should it be required again. When the procedure is complete and the child is lifted into the sitting position, signaling that the "battle" is over, he or she will probably now stop crying. One can then try to persuade the child to admit to all present that "it didn't really hurt." Even though he or she may still remember the whole procedure as total chaos, the child may also remember admitting to his or her parents that "it didn't hurt." This may result in a more sedate episode when the sutures are removed or when the child requires another minor procedure of some sort.

Recognizing Serious Disease

Serious disease in children frequently progresses very rapidly; a child who is only slightly ill may become very ill in a short time. For this reason it is particularly important to detect a potentially serious condition early in its course. However, early detection may be very difficult because the signs of illness in the early stages of many diseases in infancy and childhood can be very subtle and obscure. One can add to this the difficulty in obtaining an accurate history from a 6-month-old baby or problems encountered in examining the abdomen of an hysterical 5-year-old child who insists on keeping his or her arms around mother's neck. Consequently, one cannot help but wonder how serious pediatric disease is ever diagnosed at a stage when it can be readily treated.

In spite of the listed difficulties in diagnosing serious disease in the young child, it is usually quite possible to do so provided one remembers to look for it. Indeed, children have an advantage over adults in this regard. For example, an adult with an acute abdomen may have any one of 10 or 15 different serious illnesses. On the other hand, for the young child who has not had previous abdominal surgery, there are really only two important acute abdominal conditions that merit concern, namely appendicitis and intussusception, and to a large extent these two are age-related. Indeed, when seeing an infant or young child for the first time for any complaint, ask yourself, "What is the one serious diagnosis to be considered in this situation for a child of this age?" There is usually only one (rarely two) condition that merits serious consideration; not until this prime diagnosis is ruled out is it time to consider the other possibilities.

The infant who has been awakened from sleep intermittently with cramps for several hours should be considered to have an intussusception until one can satisfactorily exclude it. The 6-year-old who has had abdominal pain and vomiting and whose pain is now worse with movement must be assumed to have appendicitis before anything else. The 13-year-old girl who is otherwise well but limps and has pain in the groin when she jumps or runs needs to have her femoral capital epiphysis assessed before any further exercise is permitted. The 4-year-old who has had an acute febrile illness for 6 to 8 hours associated with a very sore throat and now drools must be treated as having epiglottitis until this diagnosis can be confirmed or ruled out. Serious medical disease, such as meningitis or meningococcemia, should be added to the list as well. Children do not arrive labeled "surgical' or "medical," and the physician's mind must be open to both.

With few exceptions, serious disease in children can be confirmed or ruled out by the use of simple measures. The reason for missing the important and serious diagnosis is usually failure to think of it, not lack of understanding or knowledge. Whatever the clinical situation, remembering to consider the one serious disease which pertains to that specific situation should go a long way toward eliminating major risk of missing serious disease.

Finally, one must continue to "think serious" in spite of the "he's got it, too" syndrome. Too readily is appendicitis missed in the child with abdominal pain because the child is assumed to have the same intestinal "flu" his or her siblings have or that cabin-mates at camp have. Illness in family or close contacts is significant, and knowledge of it can be very useful in reaching a diagnosis. However, too often, with unfortunate consequences, is the assumption made that a child who also becomes symptomatic must have the same condition that his or her chums do.

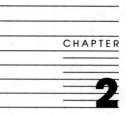
Radiology Consultations

General Considerations

In spite of the recent proliferation of new-generation techniques of imaging designed to demonstrate internal anatomy, both normal and abnormal, with a clarity not hitherto envisaged, conventional radiography continues to play a big part in emergency diagnosis. For this reason information designed to help the practitioner select the appropriate films and generally acquire more of a pediatric orientation when using this modality of investigation is included in this section.

All radiologic examinations are a subtle form of trauma. Because of this and to maintain a discriminating diagnostic judgment as well as in the interests of fiscal responsibility, the ready access to radiographic facilities that most physicians enjoy must not be abused.

Although as yet the full extent of the damage caused by ionizing radiation is unknown, it cannot be ignored. A routine skull examination delivers about one cGy to a child's eyes, and, although children's eyes are probably more resistant to radiation than the eyes of most animals, it has been shown experimentally that 15 cGy may cause lens opacities in some species. Other organs that are known to be particularly vulnerable are the thyroid gland and the gonads. The dose of radiation administered for all head, spine, and pelvic examinations is high, much higher than is required for the examination of the extremities or the chest. This must be weighed against the possible benefit when such films are being considered.

If a planned radiographic examination, or any diagnostic test for that matter, is unlikely to influence the diagnosis or change the course of the illness or its management, one needs to question its justification, not only because of the radiation dosage, but also from the point of view of providing good quality, discriminating medicine. On the other hand, a specific radiographic study should not be omitted if there is a reasonable chance of its providing information that is of value in the diagnosis or if it is likely to have a bearing on treatment.

Practical Issues

A request for a radiographic examination carries with it a request for a radiologic consultation; to permit the consultant to provide the best opinion possible, background medical information is necessary.

A brief history is very important. "Thrown from bicycle" is inadequate unless "landing on right hand" is added. "Fall" does not indicate whether the child fell down two steps or from a fourth-floor window. A chest radiograph can be interpreted much more intelligently if the radiologist knows that the child has severe asthma underlying the acute condition.

It is equally important to provide a brief outline of the relevant physical findings as well as a provisional diagnosis if one can be reached. The site of tenderness on an injured extremity tells the radiologist where to find the fracture, if one exists. A policy of recording the provisional diagnosis on the radiograph requisition not only assists the radiologist, but also induces the physician to assess the patient carefully enough to enable a provisional diagnosis to be reached.

If there is some doubt about the most appropriate examination to be selected, the radiologist or the radiology technologist should be consulted. Both are experienced professionals and are likely to have seen similar problems previously.

Extremities

In general, a suspected fracture should be splinted properly before the patient is sent to the radiology department to avoid further displacement and to alleviate pain. Sometimes, however, examination makes it clear that although a fracture is present, it is quite stable and needs no external immobilization prior to radiography. This should be a definite decision and not left to chance.

It is important to identify carefully the area to be examined. A coned view of a joint provides better detail of that joint than does a radiograph of the adjacent bone that happens to include the joint in question. A foot radiograph does not include a satisfactory view of the ankle, and an ankle radiograph does not display the foot properly. A radiograph of the tibia and fibula includes the whole tibia and fibula but does not give a good view of either knee or ankle. Similarly an injury to the distal forearm requires views of the radius and ulna, not of the adjacent wrist, as is so often requested because the child "hurt his or her wrist."

Comparison views of the opposite extremity are not warranted as a routine except for the hips, in which case they are always ordered.

Shoulder

Radiographs of the shoulder in children are often very difficult to interpret because of the large number of epiphyses. Fortunately the shoulder is rarely dislocated in children. The most common fracture in the area involves the lateral end of the clavicle. A comparison view of the opposite shoulder may rarely be helpful but should be requested only after careful reading of the initial films still leaves doubt.

Elbow

The routine views for an elbow are anteroposterior and lateral views. The anteroposterior view is taken with the joint in as much extension as is feasible and, ideally, with the forearm in supination, whereas the lateral view is best taken with the elbow flexed to 90 degrees. If there is an effusion or much soft tissue swelling about the elbow or if there is strong clinical indication of a fracture and the routine views are not diagnostic, they may be supplemented by two oblique views. The uncertainty caused by an epiphysis simulating a fracture can often be resolved by consulting a reference volume showing the normal variation in the appearance of elbow radiographs at different ages. Typical "pulled elbows" do not need radiographs.

Comparison views are warranted only after careful viewing of the initial films by someone experienced in pediatric trauma.

Forearm

Care should be taken that anteroposterior and lateral views of the forearm are not actually an anteroposterior view of the radius and ulna, combined with a film that displays an anteroposterior view of the ulna with a lateral view of the radius. These are obtained by taking the anteroposterior view with the arm fully supinated and the lateral view of the radius with the arm in the midposition. To obtain proper radiographs in two planes at 90 degrees to each other, the forearm should not be rotated between exposures.

Wrist

Wrist radiographs are not often indicated in pediatric practice. Injuries of the distal forearm warrant radiographs of the forearm bones, not of the wrist. Injuries of the carpus itself are very unusual in children. Scaphoid fractures are sometimes seen but rarely in children under age 12.

Hips

Routine examination of the hips includes anteroposterior and frog-leg (lateral) views of both hips. However, in neonates suspected of having congenital dislocation, a single anteroposterior view usually gives all the needed information. The gonads should be screened on all except one of the pelvic exposures.

Femur

The clinical diagnosis of an acute fracture of the femoral shaft requires traction immobilization of the fracture before any radiographs are taken.

Knee

The usual radiographic examination of a knee consists of an anteroposterior view of both knees and a lateral view of the knee in question. For the patella a special "skyline" view may be added, and a "tunnel" view is useful if a loose body is suspected. The lateral view of the knee is often used to confirm the diagnosis of Osgood-Schlatter disease. However, this diagnosis should be made more on clinical grounds than radiographic, and radiographs are usually not even needed in making the diagnosis.

Skeletal Survey

A skeletal survey is occasionally requested in the emergency department to detect the healing fractures and diastased cranial sutures that are so characteristic of prior child abuse. In neonates or small infants, a single "babygram" can survey the whole body.

Chest

In a routine chest examination, posteroanterior and lateral films are obtained, although in some very sick patients it may be possible only to obtain a single anteroposterior view. Children suspected of foreign body aspiration should have inspiratory and expiratory anteroposterior views as well as the lateral view. In smaller or uncooperative children, right and left decubitus films may give the same information more easily. Further information may be obtained through fluoroscopy if required. Oblique films of the chest require specific indications and are rarely necessary.

Airway

Although a soft tissue lateral view of the neck can help in the diagnosis of epiglottitis, radiographs are contraindicated in the presence of the airway obstruction which occurs with typical acute epiglottitis. Radiographs are also of little help in patients with croup, who are better evaluated clinically in most instances.

A fish bone or a fine chicken bone can only rarely be demonstrated in the pharynx or upper esophagus. When suspected, the child is best referred to the otolaryngologist for a complete examination, which will likely include endoscopy.

A retropharyngeal abscess is usually better diagnosed clinically because the normal retropharyngeal space seen in an expiratory film can be easily mistaken for an abscess. Airway views in children with prolonged stridor may reveal cervical mass lesions.

Head

The Skull Routine

Radiographs of the skull are frequently ordered after trauma when one may suspect the presence of skull fractures or diastasis of sutures. Nevertheless, it should be realized that skull radiographs are not a substitute for good neurologic assessment. In a study of cranial trauma reported from the Hospital for Sick Children, only 15 percent of 223 children with subdural hematomas had skull fractures. In addition, in 139 infants under 6 months old who had skull radiographs for cranial trauma, only 7 percent had fractures. It is clear that the presence (or absence) of a linear skull fracture without associated clinical abnormality is of questionable importance. On the other hand, depressed fractures are important, and skull radiographs are essential for their evaluation.

Skull radiography requires such positioning and restraining that the procedure is difficult for the technologist and may be very distressing for the child, particularly for a small baby. Parents have been known to withdraw their child from the radiography room midway through the procedure because of the apparent distress inflicted on the child.

For all these reasons, and in recognition of potential radiation effect, skull radiographs should be requested only if strongly indicated and not because the physician thinks that all bumped heads need radiographs.

The most useful sign suggesting the value of radiographs is an enlarging hematoma under the scalp. In such instances a fracture, if present, will almost always be located deep to the hematoma.

Facial Bones

Radiographs of facial bones should be requested if facial or orbital fractures are suspected because the routine skull radiographs do not display these bones well.

Temporomandibular Joint

Although there are special views designed to demonstrate the temporomandibular joint, they can usually be visualized satisfactorily on mandibular views.

Spine and Pelvis

Cervical Spine

If a neck fracture is suspected, the neck should be held in the neutral position and an initial cross-table lateral film of the cervical spine, down to C7, obtained. This radiograph must be read before any other studies are carried out.

Thoracolumbar Spine

A patient who may have a severe thoracolumbar spinal injury should be carefully placed on a firm radiolucent stretcher by a sufficient number of people to apply traction to the head and legs and to provide support for the spine during the transfer. A lateral radiograph is then obtained and assessed before proceeding further.

Pelvis

Radiographs of the pelvis and of the thoracolumbar spine are high-dosage views, particularly the lateral projections, which deliver about 2 cGy directly to the gonads. Hence they should be ordered only if indications are definite.

Abdomen

Routine views of the abdomen are an anteroposterior supine view and an anteroposterior upright view, although occasionally the condition of the patient does not permit the upright view. In special circumstances a lateral film may be useful, but because it entails much more radiation than the 150 mrad received during an anteroposterior exposure, there should be good reason for the additional examination before it is requested. Similar concerns apply to the right or left lateral decubitus views, although here the radiation is much less.

Skin and Subcutaneous Tissue

Abrasions

Abrasions are very common and rarely require medical help. They are the result of scrape damage to surface skin layers in addition to the effect of the friction burn. Abrasions that are superficial and harbor no embedded dirt heal rapidly and uneventfully with no permanent sequelae. Repeated application of a topical antibiotic ointment will minimize crusting and encourage healthy epithelialization without infection.

The majority of deeper abrasions heal uneventfully also, although some do result in permanent scars, especially if the child customarily forms hypertrophic scar tissue in response to superficial wounds. Very gentle washing and repeated applications of an antibiotic ointment will help to ensure optimum outcome. Rarely a deep and dirty abrasion covers such a small, well-localized area that excision and primary closure may lead to a more desirable result.

An abrasion-laceration is a common lesion in childhood, occurring often when a child has fallen on cement. Knees and chins are common sites for this injury, and the abrasion results in difficulty in repairing the laceration because the wound edges can be so gouged and shredded that simple suture is impossible. In these instances excision of the whole lesion is the method of choice, provided the area is small enough that there is sufficient tissue to pull together into a primary closure (Fig. 3–1).

All particles of dirt embedded in abraded skin must be removed to prevent permanent and disfiguring tattooing. Although one can often pick small specks of dirt out of an abrasion with the end of a scalpel, scrubbing with a surgical scrub brush is more appropriate when there are many particles of dirt. Although this is often possible without anesthesia, infiltration with a local anesthetic agent may be warranted. Satisfactory anesthesia may be obtained through topical application of 4 percent tetracaine ointment. If the child has an as-

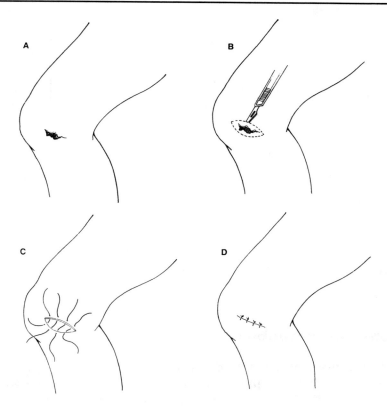

Figure 3–1 Total excision of an abrasion-laceration. Jagged laceration (A) in area with sufficient skin mobility to permit total excision (B) and primary closure (C) and (D).

sociated injury requiring general anesthesia for management, such as a forearm fracture needing reduction, the tattoo should be scrubbed clean while the child is under the same anesthetic.

Attention to the immunization status and tetanus prophylaxis is as important after a minor abrasion as it is after a laceration.

Cia Gao.   "Cia gao" is a traditional folk remedy within the Vietnamese culture. When a child has a fever, it is the custom of some Vietnamese to use coins or spoons to rub vigorously in strips on the back, chest, and neck of the child. This is thought to release some noxious matter that is the cause of the fever. Abrasions are produced that have a very characteristic and peculiar linear orientation. These are clearly due to nonaccidental trauma, and before these traditions became known in the Western world some Vietnamese refugee parents were charged with child abuse. The importance of an awareness of this condition is not so much to ensure appropriate treatment, for these lesions heal rapidly if no further trauma occurs, but to avoid the accusation of abuse. Such parents are trying to do their best in the interest of their child, and the course one should take is understanding and tactful education.

Bites

General Considerations

Wounds produced by biting, by domestic or wild animal or by another human, require careful application of the same principles of wound care as are applied to any contaminated wound. The special feature of a bite wound is heavy contamination by oral pathogenic organisms characteristic to the specific biting animal. Care of the wound must take this contamination into consideration.

Other concerns that attend the management of an animal or human bite wound include cosmetic importance and the influence this has on the choice of treatment as well as the risk of related specific infections, such as rabies or tetanus. With nonhuman bites assessment of the risk of rabies is a crucial matter.

Management Considerations

Surgical Approach to Treatment

Traditionally, the basic recommendation for management of bite wounds is to treat them open and permit healing by secondary intention. The consequence of infection after primary closure of a heavily contaminated bite wound can be disastrous, and management plans other than open treatment require careful consideration and, in most instances, consultation before being embarked on. When a bite wound is treated "open," it is packed with saline-soaked gauze, or with petrolatum (Vaseline) gauze, and covered with a bulky bandage. The packing material is gradually removed as the wound heals.

However, it is now accepted that most bite wounds can be closed safely if managed carefully by the use of established principles of care for dirty wounds. This entails copious irrigation of the depths of the wound and careful and complete debridement of wound edges and any other damaged tissue, followed by suture closure, during which as little foreign material is left in the wound as is compatible with satisfactory closure. Antibiotic coverage is customary also, although it is ancillary to proper surgical care of the wound.

Facial bite wounds or deep bite lacerations that are of the nature of incisions should all be repaired primarily within a very few hours of the incident. Although debridement of facial lacerations should be minimal, careful trimming of the wound edges and primary closure by an experienced operator usually give excellent results.

Bites caused by long, sharp, canine teeth tend to leave punctures with small superficial openings. These punctures deserve great respect and should not be closed primarily. Careful irrigation is worthwhile if it is possible. A drain inserted the depth of the puncture may prevent a spreading infection and will permit healing of the wound by secondary intention as the drain is gradually removed. When there is the slightest possibility that the puncturing tooth has penetrated deeply to violate a tissue space, tendons, or a joint, immediate referral for consideration of exploration is indicated.

One bite wound that is particularly treacherous is the injury sustained when an aggressor's clenched fist forcibly meets a victim's teeth. This punch laceration is located over the metacarpophalangeal joint, which it may enter. When the fingers extend subsequent to the incident, the access route to the joint becomes hidden under the upper wound edge, and the serious nature of the wound may not be recognized. All such wounds require open exploration and cleansing in the formal operating room suite.

Operator's Technique

The mechanical techniques employed in repair of contaminated wounds should be as gentle and atraumatic as possible. Forceps should have fine teeth to avoid compression and contusion of wound edges. Skin hooks are useful in retracting and in stabilizing a laceration as it is sutured. Closure under tension must be avoided because anything that jeopardizes blood supply facilitates growth of the pathogens within the tissue. Pressure hemostasis during the procedure or afterwards by means of the dressing as well as elevation is important because accumulation of blood within the wound increases the chance of significant infection.

Suture Material

When any heavily contaminated wound is repaired primarily, as little suture material or other foreign matter should be left within the wound as is consistent with proper wound closure. However, when the experienced surgeon carefully excises a wound, it becomes much safer to leave foreign material within its depths, and such wounds will usually tolerate formal closure in layers using absorbable material.

Sutures should be of monofilament material. There are interstices within braided sutures where organisms can flourish and low-grade infection can be perpetuated.

Antibiotics

Immediate administration of the appropriate antibiotic, prior to starting surgical repair, in full clinical dosage and by a route that gives effective blood levels quickly, is believed to decrease risk from infection locally and certainly systemically. On the other hand, antibiotics must never be used to justify a less aggressive surgical management plan. Proper surgical wound care is fundamental and must not be influenced by the availability of effective antibacterial agents.

Human oral pathogens are a mixture of gram-positive and gram-negative organisms as well as oral spirochetes. Animal saliva contains a similar variety of bacteria but also grows *Pasteurella multocida* as the main oral pathogen.

Follow-up

A contaminated wound should be checked within a day or so after repair, so it can be opened and drained if infection has developed.

Rabies

The main concern after an animal bite, apart from proper treatment of the wound itself, is the risk of rabies and the possible need for prophylaxis against rabies. Rabies is, without exception, fatal, and all effort possible must be directed toward removing any risk of a patient acquiring the disease. As serious as rabies is, it has an incubation period sufficiently long to permit active immunization against the disease during incubation, provided appropriate measures are started promptly.

Rabid animals shed the virus through saliva, and whenever a child is exposed to animal saliva, consideration must be given to the risk of rabies. This applies to bites, licking of mucosa or an open skin lesion, and scratches as well as coughs or sneezes into the subject's face. Because the animal itself may be in the prodromal stage of the disease and may still not display any overt abnormality at the time of the encounter, incarceration and observation of the animal will be necessary in many instances.

When the rabies virus enters the subject's tissues, it makes its way to the central nervous system along peripheral nerves. Therefore, the infecting agent will reach the brain sooner from a wound of the face than from a distal wound on an extremity. For this reason preventive measures are started sooner and are more aggressive for bites nearer to the head.

Dogs and cats have long been known to acquire rabies, although vaccination of domestic pets is almost routine and has greatly decreased the incidence of canine and feline rabies. Currently farm animals, including horses, cattle, sheep, goats, and pigs, are more frequent sources of the virus.

In rabies-endemic areas the wild animal population generally is the chief reservoir for rabies and is usually responsible for infection of farm animals. Foxes, skunks, and less commonly raccoons are the chief wild animals involved. Experimental attempts are being made to reduce the reservoir of rabies in this group by distributing in the appropriate habitat meat bait containing oral rabies vaccine. Unfortunately any beneficial result of this program may take years to be manifest.

Bats are also frequently infected with rabies, and any bat that bites must be considered rabid.

Rodents rarely harbor the rabies virus, although there have been rare reports of its occurrence in both muskrat and field mouse. There has not as yet been any need for concern about squirrels, chipmunks, rabbits, gerbils, and guinea pigs; a domestic pet mouse or rat who has never been out of the cage and in contact with outside animals warrants no concern about the risk of rabies.

When a biting animal, whether a pet or farm animal, has been apprehended and can be watched in incarceration, there is no need to begin antirabies prophylaxis immediately unless the animal displayed obvious illness or abnormal behavior. An animal that appears well but is shedding virus will be manifestly ill within a very few days and near death from full-blown rabies in 8 to 10 days. Hence apparent good health after incarceration for 10 days establishes that the animal did not have rabies at the time of the incident. On the other hand, if the biting animal shows signs of illness at the time of biting or during the period of observation, it should be sacrificed immediately and the brain examined at the nearest government rabies detection laboratory, where the study can usually be completed within 1 or 2 days. Any suspicion of abnormal behavior or illness on the part of the animal warrants starting antirabies treatment at once. The treatment course can be completed if the study reveals rabies virus or discontinued if it does not.

When a wild animal, such as a fox, is the biter, and it has been caught or shot, it should be killed and the head submitted for immediate study. If the animal demonstrated clear indication of abnormal behavior or illness at the time of the biting incidence, prophylaxis should be begun immediately and the full course completed if the brain study is positive.

More difficult decisions are required when the biting animal, wild or domestic, has run off and cannot be located. The following types of information are used to assist in this situation:

1. *Provocation.* A description of the incident should be obtained. An attack that was provoked by the child, who may have been teasing the animal or trying to take its food, is not characteris-

tic of the rabid animal. On the other hand, when a normally friendly dog is unusually irritable or snaps at the child without warning or reason to do so, rabies should be suspected.

2. *Behavior.* When a fox is seen prowling through an inhabited area, it should be considered abnormal. Alteration of gait or apparent confusion should suggest illness.
3. *Endemicity.* Knowledge of the incidence of animal rabies in an area is very important. Where there is no reported animal rabies one will tend not to treat unless there is clinical indication of illness in the animal.
4. *Species.* A fox or skunk is much more likely to be carrying the virus than a squirrel.

Rabies Prophylaxis

Proper wound care is the first stage in rabies prevention. Washing the wound with soap and water is effective. Quaternary ammonium solutions and antiseptics in general help to eradicate the virus from the wound.

Passive immunity is provided by the use of human immune rabies serum. Whenever vaccine is indicated, use of passive immune measures is indicated as well. When the biting animal is under observation, immediate antisera is frequently used in the interim until a decision is made regarding the need for vaccine. This measure would be particularly appropriate for facial wounds, when there is greater urgency for initiation of prophylaxis.

Active immunization is possible by virtue of the long incubation period of the disease. The vaccine used is the human diploid cell vaccine, which has little of the risks and complications that in the earlier vaccines frequently influenced too greatly the decision to immunize or not. Not only is there a greatly decreased incidence and severity of complications from the new vaccine, but also the course of injections is much shorter and better tolerated. No longer does concern about toxicity of or host reaction to the vaccine weigh heavily in the judgment required when deciding on the need for vaccination.

Tetanus Prophylaxis

The same need for evaluation of the immune status of the child is present as exists in relation to any laceration. If the child has not been given tetanus toxoid within the last 5 years, it is recommended that a booster be given.

Burns

General Considerations

The variety of causes, location, size, and depth so characteristic of external wounds generally is no less a feature of burns. The history of the burning incident itself is important in satisfactory assessment of both lesion and child and in planning management. Knowledge of how burns are produced is the basis for attempts at prevention.

A number of specific considerations arise from the history of the incident. For burns sustained in a hot water bath, the temperature of the water and the duration of exposure are significant. For higher temperatures of water, a few additional seconds of exposure can result in much greater tissue damage. Turning down the output temperature on the water heater to 130°F (54.5°C) markedly diminishes risk to tissue.

Burns sustained by contacting stove elements can be deep but do not cover a large area. A burn caused by spilled tea or coffee usually covers a significant area on the head, face, chest, and shoulder but is not often of serious depth. Sunburns can cover wide areas and result in significant systemic effect but are rarely other than first degree or superficial second degree in depth. Corrosive materials such as acids or strong alkalis often cause burns in the area of contact that are deep second degree or third degree.

Electrical burns are unique problems and usually result when the young child puts in the mouth the plug of a lamp that has been partly pulled out of the extension cord outlet into which it has been plugged. Saliva completes the contact and conducts the current to the surrounding tissue. Burns from lightning or other sources of high voltage do occur rarely, and in these instances wounds of entry and of exit are usually both discernible. The energy that passes into the tissues in these incidents may cause necrosis of deeper tissues, including bone.

As should be the policy with any traumatic injury, the physician is obligated to consider the presence of specific related injuries as complicating factors. When a flame burn involves the face, particularly if there is soot or carbon on the lips, an airway burn must be suspected. Any house fire incident, whether burns have been sustained or not, should lead one to suspect smoke inhalation. Any electrical burn, particularly if there are separate wounds of entry and exit of the current, warrants careful assessment of cardiac function because cardiac arrhythmias, especially of ventricular origin, may result from the passage of electrical current through the body.

Burns are coming to be recognized more often as the manifestation of intentional abuse. Burns restricted to the buttocks that are attributed to excessively hot bath water must draw suspicion. Children step into the hot bath before they sit down in it. Burns on the hands or buttocks of the configuration of stove elements often result from the child's hands being held on the stove or the child being held seated on the stove. Cigarette burns produce discrete, rounded, blistered spots, which can be easily mistaken for the lesions of bullous impetigo.

Investigation into the pathology of burns has revealed that heat in the burned tissues soon passes into and damages the adjacent tissue also. Progression of burn injury can be minimized if the whole region is immediately cooled off. Therefore, it is recommended that cold water be applied to a burned area, either by way of immediate splashing of water on the burn as a first aid measure or by the application of cold, wet packs to a still painful burn when a child arrives in the emergency department. An additional benefit from this cooling is its analgesic effect.

The general effects of burns have been the focus of a great deal of research over the years. When the burn area measures more than 15 or 20 percent of body area, extensive fluid loss into the burn and adjacent tissues rapidly depletes intravascular fluid. In the presence of a large area burn, small vessels generally throughout the body become abnormally permeable because of a circulating humoral factor. Maintenance of blood volume and tissue hydration becomes the basis for the medical management of the patient. Formulas designed to guide fluid replacement therapy have been derived from body weight and the proportion of body surface area covered by burn. These formulas are important clinical tools but remain in the category of guides to management. It is still necessary to follow the patient's clinical state, vital signs, and urine output.

Evaluation of the status of the patient's tetanus immunization is also required when a child is seen with a burn of any degree of seriousness. The same measures are necessary as are needed after a laceration.

Treatment

A first-degree burn, or one appearing as an area of erythema only, usually needs no specific treatment, although cool, wet packs initially may be necessary to control pain.

A second-degree burn, one with blisters, damages the superficial layers of skin, resulting in fluid accumulation between the layers. For a small burn these blisters act as an efficient dressing and need not be debrided. When the blister is large, floppy, and at risk of early rupture, it is probably worthwhile to debride the blister, excising as much of the dead tissue as is easily done. The dressing should have a greasy layer in contact with skin, covered with saline-soaked gauze, which is in turn covered with a bulky outer layer of gauze pads, all held in place with gauze bandages. Any such burns involving the face, hands, feet, or genitalia warrant consideration for plastic surgical referral because of the potential for complications from burns in these areas. Streptococcal infection can convert the damage from a superficial second-degree burn to that of a deep second-degree burn with the attendant greater risk of significant scarring. Because of the particular significance this has for a facial burn, some physicians treat all second-degree facial burns with penicillin whether hospital admission is required or not.

Children whose burns are dressed and followed on an ambulatory basis should be seen again within 2 or 3 days. The dressing should be taken down to the level of the petrolatum layer on the skin, which itself need not be removed if there is no evidence of infection. Parents should be instructed to bring the child back immediately if the dressing develops an odor or becomes discolored with exudate, or if the child develops systemic indications of infection. Concern regarding parents' ability to follow instructions is additional reason for recall in 2 or 3 days.

Burns that cover more than 10 to 12 percent of body surface area should be referred for admission because intravenous therapy will probably be needed for treatment of the systemic effects. This threshold could be a trifle higher for a healthy 12-year-old child but lower for a neonate or an older child with an underlying chronic disease. While awaiting the consultant, the child should be covered with a clean sheet and an intravenous infusion should be started.

Ideally cannulation of a vein either through stab or by cutdown should be done through intact skin to minimize the risk of infection compromising the infusion. However, in the presence of a burn covering much of the patient, it may be necessary to begin the infusion through burned skin, in which case one should not hesitate to do so. A cutdown carried out through an area of third-degree burn will require anesthesia only for the deeper layers or perhaps not at all.

Any burn, no matter how small, which is blanched, insensitive to needle prick, or charred, and therefore almost certainly third degree or full thickness, warrants referral. Not only might primary excision be the treatment of choice, but also careful assessment of the viability of underlying structures is indicated.

In severe house fire or gasoline flame incidents, circumferential third-degree burns of the chest can occur. Within a day or so these result in tough eschar formation around the chest that can seriously compromise respiratory movement. It may be necessary to incise the eschars longitudinally on both sides of the chest to permit respiratory movement. Escharotomy may also be needed on an extremity to permit its expansion if viability is compromised. Fashioning these escharotomies requires no anesthesia because the necrotic skin is totally insensitive.

When arranging to accept in referral a patient with a major burn, the main considerations to be dealt with over the telephone are (1) proper protection of airway if there is the slightest possibility of smoke inhalation or that the airway itself may be burned; (2) adequate parenteral fluid administration, especially if the transfer will take an appreciable length of time; and (3) the need for escharotomy.

Assessing Burn Area

Several rules of thumb have been devised to facilitate calculating the percentage of the body surface area that is burned. Only the part of the burn that is at least second degree is included in the calculations of fluid requirement. Parts of the burn that are erythematous alone are not included. The most useful of these methods is the "rule of nines," which is, of course, approximate but gives useful guidance in assessing a patient and planning treatment.

The rule of nines assigns 9 percent or multiples of 9 percent of the body surface area to each portion of the body, as follows: trunk, 18 percent each for front and back surface (36 percent total); legs, 9 percent each for front and back surface of each leg (18 percent per leg, 36 percent total); arms, 9 percent total for each arm (18 percent total);

1st degree erythema ▥   2nd degree ▤   3rd degree
not to be included

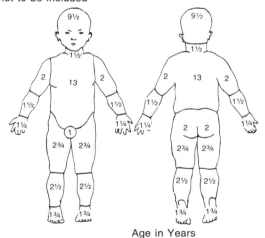

Figure 5–1 Estimation of burn area. (From Abelson WH, Smith RG. Residents Handbook of Pediatrics. 7th ed. Toronto: BC Decker, 1987:p 567.)

Area	0	1	5	10	15	Adult
Head area	19	17	13	11	9	7
Trunk area	26	26	26	26	26	26
Arm area	7	7	7	7	7	7
Thigh area	5½	6½	8½	8½	9½	9½
Leg area	5	5	5	6	6	7

Age in Years

Total 3rd degree burn_____
Total 2nd degree burn_____   TOTAL BURNS_____

head, 9 percent total; and genitalia, 1 percent. These figures apply to the larger child or adult. For younger children or infants there are modifications in the numbers that should be kept available for referring to when needed (Fig. 5–1).

Intravenous Fluid Requirements

Because of the enormous fluid loss into burns of significant surface area, aggressive parenteral fluid administration is very important if not lifesaving. Crystalloids, colloid solutions, and blood are all used, depending on timing, severity and area of the burn, and local preference. However, with few exceptions, for the first 24 hours crystalloid solution only is recommended because at least for that period the initial capillary damage and its resultant increased permeability will permit colloid solutions to leak rapidly into the interstitial space. Subsequent infusions of plasma, albumin, dextran, or blood will be at the discretion of the admitting surgeon and will be determined partly by the course of the patient and values obtained for basic blood parameters.

In the first 24 hours the initial requirement for crystalloid solution, in milliliters, is conveniently calculated by the following formula:

4.0 ml of Ringer's lactate

×

percent of body area with second-degree and third-degree burn

×

body weight in kg

Half of this initial volume is given during the first 8 hours after the burning incident. An equal amount is infused over the subsequent 16 hours.

It should be emphasized that the first infusion volume is timed from the time of burning and not the time of hospitalization, so that not only must fluid given en route from one hospital to the referral center, or by life-support workers on the scene, be taken into account, but also the hours spent after the burn without fluid intake come out of the first 8-hour infusion period. This emphasizes the critical need to start the first venous infusion as quickly as possible.

The above fluids are to replace burn losses only and must be supplemented by maintenance requirements divided evenly over each 24-hour period. These can be given by mouth if the subject tolerates oral fluids well. However, nausea and vomiting may occur, particularly if oral fluids are forced; usually maintenance fluids need to be given by vein also, at least for the first 24 hours. A solution of two-thirds 5 percent dextrose and one-third normal saline is appropriate in most cases. The volumes are calculated from the following formula:

$$100 \text{ ml/kg for the first } 10 \text{ kg}$$

$$+$$

$$50 \text{ ml/kg for the second } 10 \text{ kg}$$

$$+$$

$$20 \text{ ml/kg for each additional kg}$$

In totaling the fluid requirements, these formulas apply to the first 24 hours. In addition, during this period the condition of the child must be continually assessed and the fluid intake adjusted accordingly. Particularly useful is the urinary output, and in large area burns catheterization may be necessary to keep track of this parameter. General guidelines for urinary output are given in Table 5–1. .

Other indications of the state of hydration need to be taken into consideration as well, including oral mucosa, tears, skin turgor, thirst, level of consciousness, pulse, and blood pressure.

After the first day more of the water intake will be by mouth. It should also be remembered that other losses, such as nasogastric suction volumes, must be replaced.

Table 5–1. Guidelines for Urinary Output

AGE	VOL (± 5 ML)	AGE	VOL (± 10 ML)
0–2 mo	15 ml/hr	3–5 yr	30 ml/hr
2–12 mo	20 ml/hr	5–8 yr	35 ml/hr
1–3 yr	25 ml/hr	8–14 yr	40 ml/hr

Frostbite

Children who play outside for prolonged periods in frigid weather completely intent on their play are susceptible to frostbite involving fingers, toes, ears, and cheeks. Street hockey in the middle of winter may produce as many instances of frostbite as minor injuries from the contact. Care must be taken to make sure babies do not remove their foot coverings or their mittens when being taken for a walk in a carriage or stroller. Frost damage to the tiny fingers of small babies can occur quickly in the cold without the caretaker even being aware that the hands are uncovered.

Pain, pallor, then numbness should alert one to the progressive stages of frost damage. Later total bloodlessness and stiffness of the tissue herald early but possibly permanent damage.

Rapid rewarming is the treatment of choice because it is believed cellular damage continues until rewarming has occurred. At very early stages warming the hand in the subject's own axilla or next to the body elsewhere is adequate. Alternatively a warm water bath at 104° F (40°C) is effective. Care must be taken not to add burn damage to frostbite damage, so the temperature of warming baths must be carefully controlled.

Frostbitten tissue must not be traumatized. This applies particularly to the tissues as they are being warmed up and afterwards. When feet are frostbitten but there is still another mile or so to walk to reach refuge, it is better to walk on the feet in their frostbitten state than to thaw them out and walk on them after they have been warmed up. Little further damage will result from walking on already frozen feet. However, feet are very susceptible to tissue damage immediately after rewarming.

As tissues rewarm, pain can be intense. This signifies return of circulation and its effect on sensory nerve endings. Systemic analgesia may be required.

Blisters may form as tissues are rewarmed, signifying some loss of adherence of cellular layers. Unopened blisters should not be broken unless they are delicate ones and likely to break very soon spontaneously. If blisters are open, gentle debridement and cleansing are indicated.

Tetanus prophylaxis should be considered. Antibiotics have frequently been used to protect warmed tissues from infection, but the benefit remains unproven.

Patients with significant cases of frostbite should be admitted for observation and tissue protection because the extent of destruction is revealed only in time.

Infections of Skin and Adnexa

General Considerations

Pyoderma of various forms, such as impetigo, is common in children and characterized by exudate-filled blisters, crusting, and the tendency to spread. The infecting organism is usually *Staphylococcus aureus* or *Streptococcus hemolyticus* or a combination of the two. The response to antibiotic therapy, either topical or systemic, is generally rapid, and surgical implications are rare.

Bullous impetigo is an unusual staphylococcal infection of skin in which discrete, pus-filled blisters are produced. These can simulate the picture of multiple cigarette burns, and, therefore, child abuse should be considered in the differential diagnosis.

Superficial herpetic infections are relatively common and usually involve fingers or toes. Herpetic whitlow is a form of cellulitis of the fingertip with overlying blisters filled with liquid that is clear or, at most, slightly cloudy. This material is sterile to bacteriologic culture but readily reveals the herpetic virus on electron microscopy. The course of this condition is one of gradual resolution, and it is not clear if drainage of the blisters and debridement of the dead skin over them help in any way.

There are several forms of infections of skin and adjacent structures that localize and have surgical implications. These are generally due to pyogenic staphylococci and tend to remain localized because of the coagulase elaborated by the organisms that stimulates fibrin clotting in the interstitial spaces. This is the basis for abscess formation.

Infections caused by *S. hemolyticus* spread progressively through tissue because of the effect of "spreading factor," or hyaluronidase, producing cellulitis, in which there is little suppuration and nothing to drain.

Cellulitis

The spreading soft tissue infection usually due to streptococci or less often staphylococcus-streptococcus combination shows diffuse margins, fails to localize or fluctuate, produces a variable but often a quite marked systemic reaction, and in many instances develops around a superficial wound, scratch, or puncture which has provided bacterial access. Treatment of cellulitis is medical; antibiotic therapy with a drug appropriate for gram-positive infections is usually quite effective. If the systemic reaction is marked, admission to the hospital for parenteral therapy is indicated. The causative organism has been cultured in some instances by aspiration from the edge of the inflamed area.

When cellulitis fails to respond rapidly to antibiotic therapy, consideration must be given to the possibility of an unusual organism, the presence of pus that requires drainage, or a foreign body that became imbedded at the initial wounding.

An important form of cellulitis of infancy and early childhood is that which occurs on the face as a result of *Haemophilus influenzae*. This is an important condition because of the significant risk of general sepsis and meningitis, and immediate and aggressive therapy with the appropriate antibiotic is indicated. Most such children require admission.

Erysipelas

Erysipelas is a very unusual condition that is a spreading infection restricted to skin which shows sharply demarcated red margins; the infection is generally due to *S. hemolyticus*. In this condition the organism has been successfully cultured in some instances by needle aspiration from the advancing margin. Response to antibiotic therapy should be prompt.

Furuncle (Boil)

A boil is a specific form of suppurative staphylococcal infection that is restricted to skin. It appears sharply demarcated from the adjacent skin, and there is little surrounding inflammation. Because of its restriction to the layers of skin itself, there is little laxity in the tissue involved and pressure builds up quickly within the boil, causing marked pain and tenderness. Usually there is little liquefaction in a boil, and its contents may exist as a solid core and be extruded as such.

Moist heat is not recommended in treatment because the maceration it produces predisposes to infection nearby. Dry heat may accelerate drainage, but heat of any form can increase pain so much that it cannot be tolerated.

Boils drain spontaneously through a central punctum and leave little or no scar. Surgical incision is contraindicated. Gentle manipulation, with lifting up of the crust; gentle pressure; and tension applied to skin may all facilitate drainage, although facial boils should not be manipulated because of the risk of central spread of organisms. Antibiotics are justified if there is systemic toxicity or if the lesion is situated in the central facial zone, which potentially drains to the cavernous sinus.

Boils occasionally occur in crops. When this situation is encountered, attention should be directed to the possibility of systemic disease (diabetes, immunologic deficiencies) or a nasopharyngeal staphylococcal carrier in the family.

Subcutaneous Abscess

The abscess that is situated deep to skin becomes more diffuse and larger than a boil and, because subcutaneous tissues are looser than the layers of skin, does not develop the pressure of a boil and is consequently less painful and tender. These lesions can develop after a bruise, in which case a hematoma has probably become infected, or subsequent to an injection. Others seem to occur without any clear avenue for entrance of organisms.

Because subcutaneous abscesses need surgical drainage at some stage, early surgical referral is warranted. Antibiotic therapy is indicated if there is significant systemic toxicity or spreading cellulitis in addition. If the child appears to be ill, admission for intravenous antibiotic therapy is advisable. Some physicians also administer antibiotics just before and for a few days after drainage to minimize risk of systemic infection resulting from the surgical manipulation.

Certain other patients, such as some with congenital cardiac lesions, require antibiotic treatment to avoid infection secondarily affecting the underlying anomaly.

Most abscesses are produced by *Staphylococcus* species, although *Streptococcus* is also implicated in some, some are mixed *Staphylococcus* and *Streptococcus*, and a few are of gram-negative causation.

Subcutaneous abscesses should be differentiated from lymphadenitis that has progressed to abscess formation. These occur in areas of lymph node aggregation and are usually subsequent to a minor infection, perhaps long resolved, in its lymphatic drainage region. Adenitis less often proceeds to suppuration and the need for surgical drainage.

Subcutaneous abscesses usually necessitate incision and drainage under general anesthesia, although some may be handled under local infiltration anesthesia of the overlying surface.

During the early stages of a developing abscess it may be difficult to differentiate between abscess and an area of cellulitis. In such cases, a period of 5 or 6 days on full dosage of an appropriate antibiotic may clarify the diagnosis. The cellulitis will usually respond dramatically, whereas the abscess will show only partial improvement in the inflammatory reaction and the mass will remain.

Carbuncles are very rare in children and suggest serious underlying debilitating or immunosuppressive illness.

Puncture Wounds

General Considerations

Puncture wounds are important because of the potential for complications far more serious than the benign appearance of the initial wound would suggest. The outcomes of these injuries are so variable that a prediction of the course which has any hope of accuracy requires a full history with emphasis on as much of the following information as can be obtained:

1. Puncturing object, including degree of contamination
2. Depth of insertion
3. Completeness of removal
4. Time since the incident
5. Clothing over the puncture site
6. State of tetanus immunization

The findings on examination, when correlated with the information obtained from the history, provide further information that is crucial. If 24 hours have passed since the incident and there is no indication of inflammation, uninfected healing is likely. On the other hand, inflammation beginning within a few hours of the wounding heralds infection, which requires specific measures. Location of the point of entry directly over an interphalangeal joint introduces risk of contamination of the joint or even foreign body retention within the joint.

A piece of a metallic foreign body, such as a sewing needle, can always be demonstrated by radiograph. One cannot easily demonstrate the tip of a rose thorn that is retained in the tissues or within a joint, although radiographic visualization of air within a joint certainly establishes that the synovium has been violated. Some foreign bodies that are of limited radiopacity can still be demonstrated on radiograph by the use of special techniques. This is particularly useful when the puncture has been produced by a shard of glass from which a fragment may have broken off.

Treatment

Most minor puncture wounds that are not situated over important structures and show no inflammation require no specific treatment, although immediate warm soaking may further enhance chances of healthy healing. Inflammation beginning hours or a day or so after the wounding incident implies infection, and the decision must be made whether to explore, to start antibiotics, or to refer the patient. If history does not suggest the risk of a retained foreign body, a short course of an appropriate antibiotic in full clinical dose is warranted if early infection is apparent. If response is not satisfactory, exploration for foreign body should be considered. If referral is being considered with a view to the need for surgical exploration, referral should be early, rather than late, and not after several courses of drugs or other measures have been tried to no avail.

For further information on the management of puncture wounds, see Chapter 40.

Embedded Foreign Bodies

General Considerations

Foreign bodies are ingested, inserted, or inhaled. They are pushed into virtually every body orifice, usually intentionally. Foreign bodies are found embedded deep to skin or fingernail or toenail or within muscle, bone, or brain. They are found within joints, the eyeball, the thoracic or abdominal cavities, and sometimes the heart itself.

The rare instances of foreign body lodgment caused by medical misadventure, such as the cutdown catheter that has traveled by vein or the gastrostomy tube from which the inner end has broken off within the gastric lumen, are omitted here. Foreign body situations involving the gastrointestinal, the respiratory, or the other organ systems are discussed in other chapters.

The basic principle underlying all cases involving a foreign body is that removal is necessary to prevent complications. However, this must be tempered with careful judgment. The tiny piece of glass known to be embedded under the skin of the foot that is neither palpable nor radiopaque is often best left alone. Most foreign bodies ingested will pass uneventfully (see Chapter 22).

Many foreign bodies are amenable to easy removal under local anesthesia. However, one must remember that the tissue distortion which is caused by anesthetic infiltration can make the search for a previously easily palpable object a frustrating and interminable procedure on which one should never have embarked. Too often failed attempts at removal under local anesthesia lead to referral for secondary exploration under general anesthesia. The prime example of this is removal of a sewing needle from the sole of the foot. Even with the use of general anesthesia, the use of image intensification fluoroscopy, and the ischemia provided by tourniquet, this procedure can be very difficult.

Foreign body cases, and the management of such, must be treated with great respect by the primary physician, and a prime tenet of treatment must remain the willingness to seek help.

When a child with an embedded splinter or other foreign body is seen, the appropriate tetanus immunization is required. See the section on lacerations for details of immunization (Chapter 10).

Many other situations dealing with foreign bodies are discussed in chapters covering specific parts of the body.

Splinters

Superficial splinters or thorns lying parallel to the skin surface and visible through it are easily removed by lifting up and laying open the insensitive superficial layers of skin with a sterile needle, thus exposing the splinter, which can then be teased out with little difficulty. This process should be painless if care is taken to keep the needle pointed parallel to the skin surface and not directed deeply at any time. The very shallow erosion thus created heals rapidly.

The small splinter or thorn that has been driven in perpendicular to the skin surface in such a way that only the end is visible can often be removed in a similar way. After some of the superficial layers of skin have been lifted off, the splinter may be grasped by fine non-toothed thumb forceps or impaled on a needle point and lifted out. Care must be taken when doing this, though, to lift directly outward so as not to break off the tip of the splinter or thorn.

Although some deeper splinters can be removed under local anesthesia, this method should be tried only if the foreign body is visible or palpable and will not be totally obscured by the infiltration of the anesthetic. A scratch or ink mark made before the anesthesia is injected helps to guide the incision.

Special care must be taken when the foreign body has entered the skin over a synovial joint. From time to time sepsis in an interphalangeal joint is shown to have been caused by intra-articular lodgment of a thorn or small splinter. Sometimes an indolent, low-grade inflammatory reaction in a small joint is shown, when exploration is carried out as a last resort, to be caused by the retention of the tip of a rose thorn.

Radiographic assessment for an embedded foreign body is often useful. Metallic foreign bodies are easily demonstrated by radiograph, whereas others with limited radiopacity, such as some types of glass, can often be visualized using special techniques. Many objects, however, have the same radiodensity as soft tissue, and a negative radiograph does not rule out retention of such a foreign body. When requesting radiographs for a small foreign body, the physician should seek advice from the radiographer, who will have carried out the study many times. Tangential views, soft tissue techniques, and taping a radiopaque marker on the overlying skin are all measures that can facilitate the demonstration and removal of a small foreign body which may not otherwise be easily visualized.

Many foreign bodies are embedded so deeply as to make exploration and removal under infiltration anesthesia extremely difficult. These situations require a carefully planned procedure under general, or alternatively, regional anesthesia, with all additional efforts to make the operation as simple and straightforward as possible. Use of a tourniquet to produce a bloodless field, positioning in the most convenient way (e.g., prone position for exploration of the sole of the foot), and fluoroscopy with image intensification facilitate finding the object. However, in spite of all measures that can be adopted to make the procedure easier, searching for a deeply embedded foreign body can be one of the most difficult and frustrating of operations and needs to be carried out as a formal operating theater procedure.

Not all foreign bodies should be surgically removed. It is meddlesome to plow through a thigh muscle looking for the tip of a needle. A small piece of glass embedded in the sole of a foot can be impossible for the physician to see or feel, and attempts at removal are often unjustified. When a small, superficial foreign body is left in place because it cannot be seen, it may work itself out, or a tiny abscess may form around it and extrusion of the foreign body may occur when the abscess drains. Sometimes the tiny object becomes encapsulated within fibrous tissue and produces no further symptoms. On the other hand, when a foreign body that is undetectable continues to produce symptoms, there is clear need for surgical referral with a view to exploration under a form of anesthesia that does not obscure the local landmarks.

Although a splinter embedded under a fingernail or toenail is known to lead to subungual infection, in most instances it is left in place because many physicians are unaware of a simple way of obtaining adequate anesthesia of the matrix. Although digital block anesthesia is quite effective in these instances, simple infiltration of the nail bed is also effective and is quicker and easier to achieve than a nerve block (Fig. 9–1). After a small area on the fingertip has been anesthetized, the area of anesthesia is extended proximally into the distal nail bed by continuing slowly and steadily to inject solution and advance the needle. The portion of nail bed that is anesthetized blanches and is readily identified in this way. Excising a V-shaped portion of nail over the anesthetized part of the matrix then exposes the splinter and permits easy removal.

Barbed Objects

When barbed objects such as fishhooks and crochet needles become embedded in or under the skin, their removal is made possible by pushing the hook on through the skin so the point with the barb can then be broken off before the main shaft is pulled back through the tissue (Fig. 9–2). This can usually be done quite easily under infiltration anesthesia. A variety of other maneuvers have been recommended that depend on withdrawal of the barb through the route of entry while attempting to shield the tissues from the barb by a knife blade or other

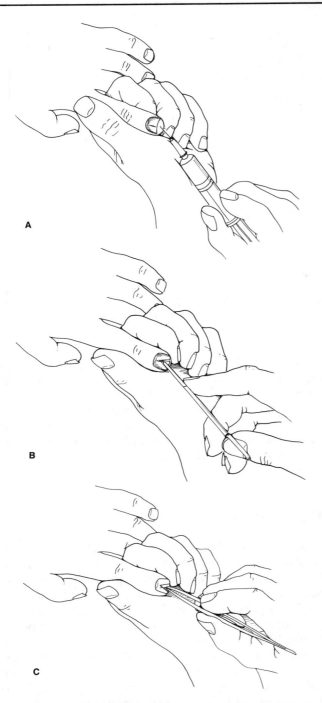

Figure 9–1 Removal of subungual splinter. *A*, Tip of finger and distal part of nail bed anesthetized by slowly injecting enough local anesthetic agent distally that it spreads proximally beneath the nail. Blanching identifies the desensitized portion of the nail bed. *B*, V-shaped portion of nail over the splinter excised with fine scissors, permitting simple removal of the splinter (*C*). Note how the instrument in use or the hand holding it is pressed firmly against the operator's left hand, which, in turn, tightly grips the patient's finger, ensuring all units move together if the affected finger moves.

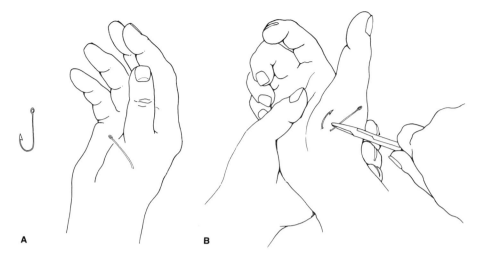

Figure 9–2 Removal of fishhook. *A*, Fishhook embedded deep to skin. After local anesthetic infiltration of the area, the hook is gripped firmly with a needle driver and forced further so as to push the hook out through the skin (*B*). The barbed end is then broken off to permit withdrawal of the hook.

instrument inserted along the shaft and held against the barb. At The Hospital for Sick Children, such attempts have not been any less traumatic than removal by advancing through the skin surface.

If the point and barb have become lodged deep in the subcutaneous plane or in an area where there is an underlying nerve, a significant blood vessel, or a joint, radiographs of the area are needed. No attempt to manipulate the object should be made prior to appropriate surgical referral.

Encircling Objects

Fingers are seen frequently that have been inserted into holes in a wide assortment of objects and for one reason or another cannot be removed. These objects are usually metallic rings, pull-tabs from cans, washers, and occasionally glass or plastic containers. Infrequently a wire or some form of metal ring or similar object is caught around a toe. Rarely, the penis has been inserted into a bottle and cannot be removed because erection has developed.

Removal of these objects from the affected member involves a variety of mechanical procedures using grease, string, wire cutters, ring cutters, and pliers. A useful metal cutter, strong enough to cut metallic rings 4 or 5 mm in thickness, is the double-action bolt cutter from the operating armamentarium of the orthopaedic surgeon. Sometimes an auto mechanic or a hospital engineer will be more suited to the mechanical challenge presented than a physician, and for unusual cases there should be no hesitation in consulting the hospital engineering service.

In the majority of instances, encircling rings can be removed with the assistance of a lubricant. Sometimes string wrapped tightly around the finger distally with the end pulled under the ring proximally will work the ring gradually down the finger when the proximal end is pulled distally (Fig. 9–3). However, at least some of these measures have invariably been attempted before the child is brought to the hospital, and it is unusual for the emergency physician to be able to remove a ring safely without cutting it. Furthermore, to minimize tissue damage it is inadvisable to prolong excessively the effort to remove a ring without cutting it, unless the patient is adamant that this be done because of special value of the ring, financial or sentimental.

The "hair-tourniquet syndrome" is a condition seen from time to time in young babies, rarely more than 2 or 3 months in age. The cause is usually unknown, although in the occasional instance the application of the hair is suspected to be nonaccidental, or a form of child abuse.

In the hair-tourniquet syndrome one or two toes are usually involved, and rarely a finger is involved. There are reports of the penis as the site; see the section on traumatic conditions of the penis (Chapter 31). There is a visible constriction around the toe, the distal part of which is swollen and very red, with the demarcation of these changes situated at the site of the constriction. Here the end of a fine hair, or thread, can sometimes be seen on close inspection (Fig. 9–4).

A blunt nerve hook or probe can be used to lift out of the constriction groove any thread or hair. It is apparent that the hair may be wound around the toe a number of times. Usually it has eroded through skin and is actually lying in the subcutaneous plane. When the hair or thread has been removed in this way, the residual lesion has the appearance of an encircling incision through skin.

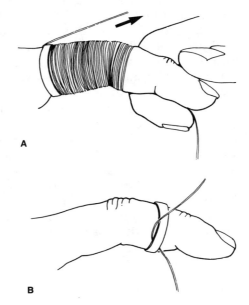

Figure 9–3 Ring removal. Showing the "string" method for removal of a tight ring from a finger. *A,* String is wound tightly around the finger, beginning distally, until the ring is encountered. Here the proximal end of the string is passed under the ring and is pulled in a distal direction as it is unwound, until the ring is forced over the interphalangeal joint (*B*), from where it is easily slipped off.

A

B

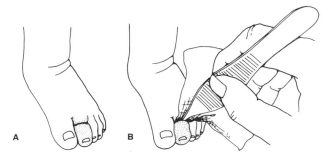

Figure 9–4 Hair-tourniquet lesion. *A*, Circumferential constriction ring visualized. *B*, Removing the deeply embedded fragments of hair or thread using forceps and sponge.

In spite of the difficulty in visualizing any foreign material in the deep constriction passing around the toe, one must persist in finding the material and removing it either by the use of the blunt hook or blunt thumb forceps or by wiping in the depths of the incision with gauze. Rapid healing follows complete removal.

Embedded Earring Butterfly

The custom to pierce the earlobe in those even as young as 1 or 2 years has increased the incidence of injury caused by an embedded earring butterfly. How the butterfly on the earring post resting against the posterior aspect of the lobe is permitted to erode into the tissue of the lobe is difficult to explain. A too-tight application coupled with neglect may be the chief causative factors.

When the baby, child, or teenager shows up in the emergency department, the complaint often is that "the earring won't pull out of the ear even though the butterfly has been missing for some time". One can suspect with this story that the butterfly is not missing at all but is still lodged firmly on the post and has gradually been pulled into the tissue of the earlobe, where it has been covered from view posteriorly by skin that seems to have grown over it. This can be readily confirmed by gentle palpation of the earlobe itself.

Removal is simple. Infiltration of the earlobe from the back with local anesthetic agent will give complete anesthesia of the entire area. A fine mosquito hemostat is used to spread widely the almost obliterated opening at the back of the earlobe and to grasp the butterfly, which is then extracted. The earring can then be removed.

The wound usually heals rapidly. No further foreign bodies should be inserted until complete healing has been achieved, and at that time the earlobe may have to be pierced again if the subject wishes to continue wearing this form of jewelry.

Lacerations and Suturing

General Considerations

In a children's hospital, the skill with which a child with a laceration
is handled is believed to be at least as important as the surgical technique. In most hospitals there will be many sources for advice.
Specialty residents and staff are often available. Therefore, if there is
any doubt as to how to proceed with a child with a laceration, one
should not hesitate to ask for help. Emergency nurses see lacerations
treated day after day, and the knowledge that they have acquired is
invaluable. The physician should take advantage of it. When an emergency nurse summons help because an inexperienced intern is having difficulty with either a laceration or the child, the nurse is merely
doing what a good emergency nurse should do.

Current trends in management include greater involvement of parents in treatment procedures such as suturing of lacerations. Although
for the first few pediatric lacerations encountered the physician may
have difficulty in giving the image of competence, familiarity with both
equipment and techniques is quickly achieved. When that stage is
reached, one should not hesitate to permit a parent to stay with a child
while a laceration is being repaired, although it is usually best to permit only one parent to attend.

Parents who insist loudly on attending are often the ones least likely to be helpful. Conversely those who do not have the aggressiveness
to demand they be admitted to the treatment room are frequently the
ones to help the most. Hence, do not hesitate to suggest that a parent
be in attendance if you feel it would benefit the child and not compromise the procedure.

Occasionally removal of a parent who is already in the suture room is the only measure that will garner some degree of cooperation from the patient. The restrained child often continues to shout to a parent to be "rescued" but may quiet down and cooperate when there is no parent visible. However, because this may seem to the child to be punishment for his or her behavior, it should be a last resort. On the other hand, a parent in attendance must understand that the physician is in charge in the suture room and may ask the parents to leave if that proves to be necessary.

One should also remember that a parent who is already visibly upset may be much more disturbed by the surgical atmosphere in the treatment room and is likely to faint. Indeed, whenever a parent is present while you are suturing, he or she should be watched closely so quick removal can be effected should any early signs of fainting be noted.

If a parent requests a specific physician to treat the child, a reasonable attempt should be made to call that physician. Let that individual be the one to indicate that he or she is not on call or cannot come; the emergency staff need not take on that responsibility. If a plastic surgeon is requested for a laceration that does not justify the consultation, tactful attempts may be made to persuade parents to be more realistic. However, if they insist on the referral, the patient should be referred, no matter how minor the laceration. If a parent is especially upset or demanding, particularly aggressive, or already complaining about quality of care, it is wise to discuss the situation with a colleague or an appropriate consultant before proceeding.

Systemic Effects

Hemorrhage, with its potential for producing hypovolemic shock, is an important early systemic manifestation potentially resulting from a laceration. However, it is important to realize that, with the exception of the uncommon severe scalp laceration, few cuts in childhood ever bleed sufficiently to cause shock. For this reason, in a child with several lacerations after a vehicular accident, probably something else is causing hypovolemia, such as a ruptured spleen. Attributing hemorrhagic shock to a fractured femur and several lacerations is a common error in childhood trauma and can lead to delay in diagnosis of the offending internal injury.

Airway compromise by blood from an intraoral laceration must also be watched for, particularly in an individual whose level of consciousness is diminished.

Infection can be a delayed complication of any open wound. However, the management of wound infections is too broad a field in itself to be dealt with here except to emphasize proper wound care and aseptic technique.

The Decision to Suture

Most lacerations are repaired primarily to speed healing, stop bleeding, and minimize scarring. Suturing is the usual method to hold a laceration closed.

Lacerations That Do Not Require Primary Suturing

Palatal or Lingual Cuts. In most instances, mucosa heals rapidly and well. An intraoral laceration should be sutured if it produces a food pocket or if a mobile flap has been raised that will be in the way as the child chews. One or two stitches are sometimes needed to stop persistent bleeding from a cut on the tongue.

Puncture Wounds. Puncture wounds that fall together do not require suturing.

Superficial Lacerations. Superficial lacerations that do not involve the deep dermis and do not gape (deep scratches) need not be sutured primarily.

Lacerations That Should Not Be Sutured

Grossly Contaminated Lacerations. An excessively dirty cut on the sole of the foot, such as one sustained in a barnyard or a grossly contaminated pond, should probably be treated open. In addition, one invites complications by closing wounds adjacent to heavily contaminated areas such as the anus. Animal bites are contaminated with oral organisms and frequently result in infection. They may be treated open in locations with little or no cosmetic importance, although most can be sutured primarily provided the wounds are irrigated copiously and properly debrided before closure. Facial wounds are always sutured.

Lacerations After Excessive Delay. Suturing is traditionally considered to be contraindicated after a delay of 12 to 18 hours, although even then suturing is often permissible, provided careful cleansing and debridement is carried out, and if it is situated in an area with ample blood supply. For wounds with high potential for contamination a delay of 6 to 8 hours may be too long.

Embedded Foreign Body. A wound should not be closed until any embedded foreign material has been removed.

Considerations for Referral

Size, Depth, Degree of Contamination, and Nature of the Cut. Involvement of deeper structures, such as tendons and nerves, requires referral. Stellate lacerations, those amid deep abrasions, and those extensive enough to require general anesthesia should be referred. A sciving, avulsing wound may need grafting. A thin flap with questionable viability and a significant defect in skin both require surgical referral. If experienced judgment is required to determine treatment for a heavily contaminated wound, surgical consultation is in order.

Location. Lacerations across the free margin of the eyelid and the vermilion border of the lip (unless a very small cut) may need to be referred. Many facial cuts, depending on direction and specific location in relation to skin lines, also may require referral.

Patient Assessment

History is important. The description of the accident may suggest the need to look carefully elsewhere for associated injuries, or it might indicate heavy bacterial contamination of the wound. A history that is vague, is inappropriate for the child's age, changes from minute to minute or when related by the second parent may suggest the possibility of child abuse. Furthermore, from the epidemiologic point of view, we want to know what causes injury because this is essential in any continuing program to prevent accidental injury.

Examination is the aspect of patient assessment most often incompletely carried out and inadequately recorded. Complete and proper examination of the injured member and adequate general examination are necessary for appropriate treatment.

Associated injuries should always be sought, especially those most likely to complicate the presenting lesion. When a child arrives with a lacerated chin after falling from a bicycle, one should look particularly for a mandibular fracture in the region of the temporomandibular joint. An eyebrow laceration requires evaluation of the eye and vision. Laceration of the wrist or palm requires careful assessment of nerve and tendon function. Furthermore, proper examination is necessary to satisfy legal requirements not only for the emergency department, but also for the physician's personal protection. The physician must not cut corners when examining the patient or when recording that examination.

Preparing to Suture

Watching the physician open the tray, fill the syringe with anesthetic material, open the suture pack, and pour the preparation solutions is almost as traumatic for the child as undergoing the procedure itself, sometimes more so. In fact, when all this is done after the child enters the treatment room, the patient rapport that the physician has tried so hard to obtain can be completely lost. All preparations should be completed before the child is brought in, down to the very last maneuver, including filling the syringe with anesthetic material and fixing the suture into the needle driver.

Suturing is a surgical procedure. If the physician is not wearing an operating theater "scrub suit," a clean gown over street clothes satisfies proper aseptic technique, although this is impractical for many emergency department situations. Although infection is mainly a result of the features of the wound itself and of the surgical care it receives, surgical mask and head covering are certainly in order, partly for the antisepsis they provide, partly to assist in the general maintenance of good aseptic policies.

Thorough hand scrubbing for every laceration is not as necessary as it is prior to every formal operating theater procedure. However, a physician who will be repairing a number of cuts during a shift should do a full preoperative hand scrub at the start of the shift and once or twice again during the shift. A brief scrub before each individual procedure should then suffice.

To minimize the risk of gram-positive infections developing in treated wounds, the physician should remain alert to the possibility of transfer of infection when dealing with patients who have apparent skin infections or streptococcal pharyngitis. When seeing these patients, the physician should wear gloves, which should then be carefully discarded. Hands should also be washed after exposure to every patient but particularly after exposure to patients with infections.

Gloves should be worn during all suturing procedures. However, they should not be put on until the physician is sure the nurse needs no further help in positioning or restraining the child.

Restraint

Although a knowledge of different techniques of patient restraint is important in carrying out minor surgical procedures in childhood, one should not restrain a child unless it is necessary. A goal that pediatric emergency personnel strive to reach is to handle as many children as possible in such a way that restraint is not needed. If one selects the child carefully, reassurance, distraction, and avoidance of pain can do wonders. Restraining a child unnecessarily is probably just as unfortunate an error in judgment as is failing to restrain a child who then requires it during the procedure.

The standard method of using a sheet to "bunny" a small child is quite effective and does not require special equipment (Fig. 10–1). More recent methods entail the use of special restraint boards, which come in several sizes and are also quite effective (Fig. 10–2). Unfortunately, in those institutions in which the manufactured restraint boards are used routinely, the nursing staff all too often forget how to bunny a child properly.

Firm restraint is also very useful when one sutures the hand of a child. Proper tape fixation of a forearm to a rigid splint permits the nurse to immobilize the arm with one hand. The time taken to apply proper limb restraint for a lacerated hand or finger is saved many times over during the procedure (Fig. 10–3).

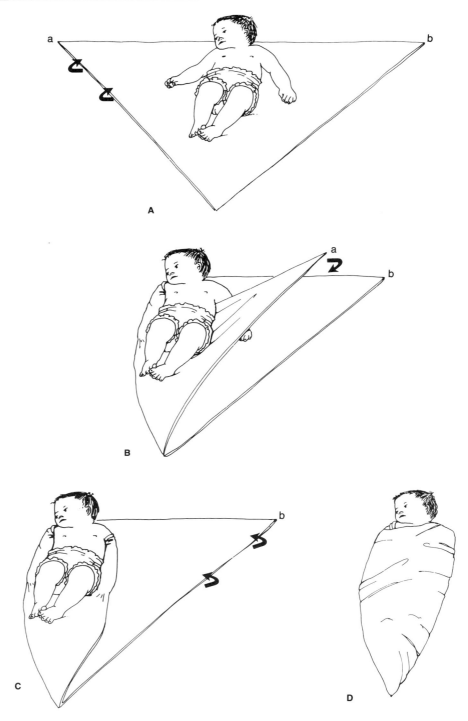

Figure 10–1 "Bunnying" a child with sheet. *A,* Initial folding of the sheet and placement of child on the sheet. *B,* One corner, "a," is wrapped around right arm, passed under child's body, and pulled tight to hold the arm securely. *C,* Remaining part of point "a" wrapped around left arm and passed back under child's body, thus holding the left arm. *D,* Point "b" is then wrapped over child and back under, completing the restraint.

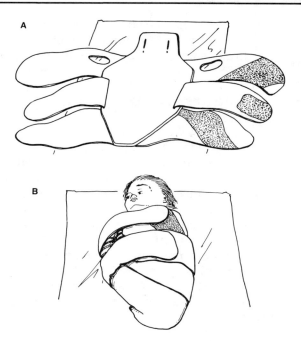

Figure 10–2 Using a restraint board. Commercially produced restraint boards of several sizes are currently available and are very effective in immobilizing a child. *A*, The board ready to be used. *B*, A child totally restrained on a board. One arm or leg can be left out if required. For the particularly vigorous child, or the one who continually manages to free one arm, restraint within a sheet followed by application of the restraint board rarely fails whatever the strength of the child.

Shaving the Wound

Eyebrows should never be shaved. Regrowth is very slow. One can usually avoid shaving the scalp. Greasing hair down with sterile petrolatum or even just wetting it down with preparation solution is often sufficient to hold it out of the way. If hair is still a major hindrance to effective wound care, cutting the hair short with scissors to 0.5 to 1 cm around a laceration may be adequate. These methods are all that are required in the handling of most scalp lacerations. Formerly, rigorous shaving was done around all scalp wounds to decrease the

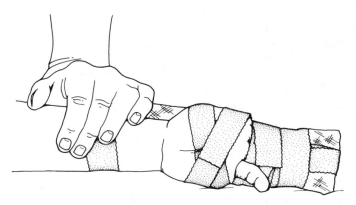

Figure 10–3 Arm immobilization. The arm and hand are taped to a splint with the finger to be treated excluded. This permits the assistant to maintain satisfactory control over the extremity by simply holding the splint with one hand.

risk of infection. The current policy of shaving only when cuts are particularly dirty, need extensive debridement, or are associated with a fracture has not led to a significantly increased incidence of infection.

Preparation, Draping, and Lighting

An antiseptic that stings excessively should never be used. Soap and water is useful on dirty skin, but remember to wash all soap from a cut. An aqueous preparation solution containing molecular iodine is customary, but its mechanical cleansing effect is probably as important as its germicidal properties. Copious irrigation of the heavily contaminated wound with saline is probably as important in preventing infection as anything else is.

When draping, one should try to duplicate operating theater techniques as closely as possible. However, it is usually best not to cover a frightened child's eyes with a towel because this will increase his or her fright and may lose for you the cooperation gained with a great deal of effort.

It is rarely necessary to shine the operating light into a child's eyes. In fact, the theater lamp is basically designed to produce illumination in a deep hole and is generally unnecessary for a facial laceration. When needed, the light can often be angled down over the face in such a way that the supraorbital ridges shade the eyes.

Local Anesthesia

Lidocaine, 1%, without epinephrine, is a standard solution for infiltration that is applicable to most lacerations. Allergy to lidocaine is rare but should be ascertained whenever one proposes to use the material.

The inclusion of epinephrine dramatically decreases bleeding and increases the safe dose of the anesthetic agent, which can be given by 50 percent or more. However, there are a number of sites where epinephrine must never be used, such as a finger, a toe, the nose, the penis, and the pinna, and in the interest of safety it probably should not be readily available for routine use.

Unless the wound is excessively dirty, the anesthetic agent should be injected directly into the superficial subcutaneous fat through the wound itself, not through intact skin. This technique is virtually painless. A very small needle should be used, preferably a No. 30, and the liquid must be injected *very* slowly. Lidocaine causes pain if it is not injected slowly; unless there are strong reasons for haste, there is no justification for injecting rapidly. After the first needle insertion all subsequent insertions should be through already anesthetized tissue. One should use enough solution to produce visible swelling and, ideally, blanching. Get complete anesthesia. Telling a child that the "freezing" will permit painless sewing and then not producing just that are not acceptable. At least half the time spent in repairing a laceration should be spent in anesthetizing. Do it slowly, meticulously, and completely.

A maximum does of up to 0.5 ml per kilogram of 1% lidocaine without epinephrine is generally safe.

Digital blocks are very useful for some lesions on fingers and toes. However, they are more difficult to do well than infiltration, and one should not embark for the first time on a digital block on a small child's finger without appropriate instruction. There are tricks that make blocks more effective, and these are learned by experience. Avail yourself of the experience of those around you.

TAC (solution of 0.5% tetracaine, 1:2,000 epinephrine, and 11.8% cocaine) is popular in some centers as a topical anesthetic agent for lacerations. A sterile gauze square soaked in the solution is folded into and over the laceration for 10 to 15 minutes prior to repair. There are good reports of the results, provided the repair is not delayed appreciably beyond the 15-minute interval. Currently we have had no experience in this modality.

Handling the Moving Target

Those who treat children soon become accustomed to extremities that do not hold still, heads that suddenly turn when somebody enters the room, and chins that move constantly. In spite of all efforts to restrain, this restlessness inevitably results in needles unexpectedly pushed in farther or pulled out, thumb forceps that pull through skin that suddenly tries to escape, and suture needles that do not end up where they are aimed. It is always a good principle to anticipate that a child will move suddenly when least expected.

One must learn how to move with the child and work on the operative site as it moves. A right-handed person does this by placing the left hand firmly on or beside the laceration and by using this hand to support and guide the injecting or suturing hand. A lacerated chin must be firmly grasped by the left fingers and thumb; this hand is then used to guide either the anesthetizing needle or the needle-driver as it is held in the operator's right hand. One should not use thumb forceps when there is risk of the wound suddenly moving because the fine-toothed forceps used in wound repair can readily pull through a small child's skin. The basic objective in this technique is to make the area of the laceration, the operator's hands, and the instrument in use all one unit, the members of which move together. Experience using this method permits satisfactory suture repair of most moving lacerations (Fig. 10–4).

In spite of all efforts taken to facilitate the treatment of lacerations in the struggling child, special measures are necessary when the wound is situated close to the eye. Every physician who sutures lacerations in an emergency department fears that someday he or she will inadvertently impale the cornea of the struggling child with a needle while anesthetizing or suturing a cut close by. As well as carefully bracing oneself against the child's head, one should always direct the nee-

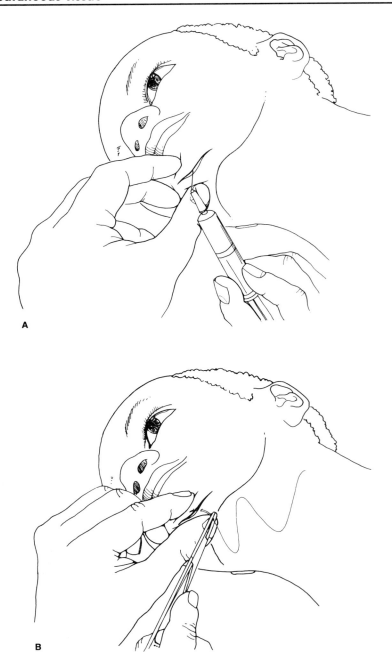

Figure 10–4 Anesthetizing and suturing the moving target. When anesthetizing a laceration on a moving chin the left hand must grip the two sides of the laceration firmly (*A*).
The syringe is pressed firmly against the left thumb, thus joining the patient, the operator's left hand, and the syringe into one unit, all parts of which move together when the
chin moves. The No. 30 needle can be bent to give optimum ease and comfort. Note
that it enters the subcutaneous fat via the open cut and does not pass through intact
skin. When suturing, the needle driver is similarly guided by the left thumb so stitches
can still be inserted even though the chin is not kept still (*B*). (Gloves should be worn
during suturing.)

dle away from the eye in such a way as to minimize the chance of ocular damage should the child suddenly look toward the operator.

Suturing

In closing wounds, aim for apposition, not strangulation. Remember, however, that knots tied loosely will become even looser as the edema caused by the anesthetic agent injected into the tissues subsides.

The suture material chosen should be easy to manipulate and remain tied. Although plastic monofilament sutures are the standard products used on the face and hands, they are often difficult for the inexperienced to use because their resilience is a hindrance and knots tend to come untied. Some physicians prefer a braided synthetic thread because it has many of the advantages of a plastic material as well as the ease of handling of silk sutures, in spite of the increased risk of infection from organisms lodged in its interstices.

Use 5–0 material on most head and neck lacerations, with 6–0 on sites of particular cosmetic importance, provided there is little or no tension. Fast-absorbing plain catgut can be used for situations in which suture removal will be particularly difficult. Other absorbable materials remain so long that removal is usually necessary anyway.

When hemorrhage is a problem, it is usually unwise to spend time catching and tying bleeders. With most lacerations persistent bleeding is best handled by prompt suture closure. Time spent calming a child down may help in this regard also because the process of settling a child down doubtless has a comparable effect on blood pressure. If the bleeding is excessive, a pressure dressing and referral is the safest course.

Debridement is needed if the tissue is torn, jagged, dirty, contused, or lacking blood supply. Dirty wound edges are better cut off than scrubbed off. If extensive debridement seems indicated, it should be handled by someone with experience, as should any facial laceration that appears to need significant debridement.

When a cut is completely anesthetized, look in its depths. You may find a foreign body that should be removed, a tendon that needs repair, or even a crack in bone.

It is usually best to use a single layer of simple interrupted stitches. Subcutaneous layers rarely need suturing and then only in the deepest of cuts. The more important the site is cosmetically, the smaller the stitches and the closer together they should be. Unsightly scars can usually be easily revised. Crosshatches from big stitches are very difficult to improve.

A clean, straight laceration, the edges of which are perpendicular to the skin margins, is advantageously repaired with a subcuticular technique if there is little tension on the wound and the operator is accustomed to the technique. Alternatively, if there is concern that a laceration repaired with the subcuticular technique might open up under the tension, several superficial interrupted subcutaneous stitches included in the repair might provide the additional strength needed. The use of synthetic tapes after suturing may help, although with small children the risk of them removing all dressings and tapes must be kept in mind.

While sewing, try to keep the skin edges everted. If they persistently tend to invert, one or two mattress stitches may be useful. These can usually be removed when all other stitches have been inserted and then replaced with simple stitches. If cosmesis is not of special importance, the stitches may be left in place. If traction on one end of the laceration lines up the edges satisfactorily, a good method is to put in an end stitch and use the ends of this stitch, left long, to apply traction to the laceration. This permits the edges to be lined up accurately.

Special key sutures are needed to close the apex of a V-shaped cut (Fig. 10–5). This involves passing the needle across the apex of the flap in the superficial subcutaneous plane, not down through it, to avoid jeopardizing the circulation of the tip. One is advised not to embark on the repair of such a laceration without knowing how to effect the closure properly.

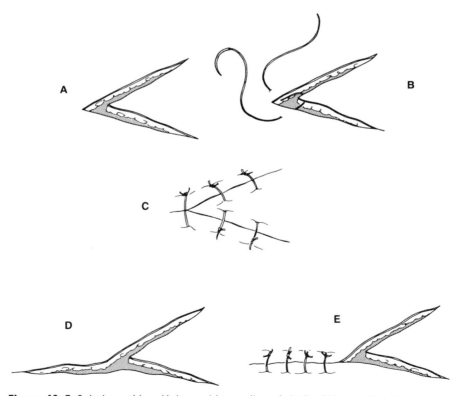

Figure 10–5 Suturing a V- or Y-shaped laceration. *A,* In the V laceration the point of the V is pulled home by a suture that passes across the tip in the subcutaneous plane (*B*), so as not to render it ischemic. *C,* The two limbs of the V are then sutured separately. *D,* In repairing a Y laceration one limb of the Y is closed (*E*), and the remaining V is repaired as above.

Leave each stitch long enough to facilitate removal but short enough to prevent its being caught in the adjacent suture. A good rule of thumb is to cut all stitches just shorter than the distance between them. If you are cutting sutures from a laceration on a child who is struggling, it is as important to form a unit consisting of patient, operator, and instruments, with everything moving together, as previously described. Hence, rest the scissors on the skin at the stitch to be cut, turn them so they are oriented perpendicular to the skin, and then cut the stitch without lifting the instrument from the child. Even with a struggling child, this permits consistent length of suture and avoids cutting the child.

Alternative Methods of Closure

Several different types of synthetic tapes are frequently used to obtain a nonsuture closure. These have been demonstrated to be effective in adults but have been less useful in children who are more apt to fiddle with dressings and are frequently able to remove all tape, gauze, and any other material that may have been applied. Because of this, it is necessary to suture many pediatric lacerations that would be suitable in adults for tape closure.

Lacerations in areas that are not of major cosmetic importance or subject to friction or pressure can be very conveniently handled by stapling. In selecting cases for stapling, though, it is necessary to choose ones that can be apposed easily and kept apposed manually while the staples are being inserted. Stapling does not close a wound as the process of tightening a suture does and, in effect, acts to hold the wound in the state it was in at the time of insertion of the staples. Scalp lacerations are the ones most often suitable for staple closure, and in this site the patient usually does not require anesthesia because the insertion of the staples is almost painless. This results in one being able to close a scalp laceration quickly and conveniently, without requiring either needles or the time involved in careful preparing and draping and anesthetizing.

Dressings

The physician must decide what the dressing is for before choosing the material to be used. Nothing may be needed; if so, nothing should be used. Moist, macerated areas, such as lip or the chin in a drooling child, are often best left open to the air. Indeed, there is a growing tendency to leave any small laceration open to the air unless there is need for protection from rubbing by clothes or hands. Hairy areas, such as scalp or eyebrow, are best left open because a dressing is not likely to stay in place anyway.

There is little scientific evidence to support the long-held general principle that covering suture lines restricts bacterial access. Certainly large extremity wounds with subcutaneous dead space or persistent oozing after repair require firm pressure dressings. Gauze squares, roller bandages, tape, and surgical dressing pads are all used depending on circumstances. On the other hand, particularly for lacerations on the head and neck, unless there is good reason for pressure or the immobilizing effect of a firm dressing, exposure probably provides the best result. Parents can often be advised to leave the laceration exposed unless the child tends to handle it, in which case they can cover it with a simple gauze dressing (i.e., Band-Aid).

If a laceration is near a major joint, it is often valuable to dress with a bulky bandage that also restricts movement. Sometimes a rigid splint or even a plaster cast may be necessary. Indeed, restriction of joint movement may be just as necessary for a few days after the sutures are removed as before when the suture material was helping to hold the cut closed.

Persistent oozing from a wound or from adjacent abrasions warrants a petrolatum dressing covered with gauze to minimize sticking of the dressing to the surface.

Antibiotic ointment is often used by some surgeons and may be applied either under a dressing or when the sutures are left uncovered. The benefit conferred by this measure is more likely because of the greasy nature of the material and resultant decrease in crusting, which makes suture removal easier and decreases the stitch marks remaining behind. An antibiotic applied to the skin surface is unlikely to influence the development of infection within the wound.

For wounds on young children who spend most of their waking hours destroying or removing bandages and tapes, it is necessary to "baby-proof" the dressing. This requires adroit use of tapes, splints, and sometimes plaster. A sleeve or pant leg may have to be pinned over a bandaged hand or foot. A sock or mitten can be applied to the hand and then pinned to the sleeve of the child's sleepers. Conversely, it is sometimes the dressing itself that aggravates the child, and leaving the wound open may be the best way to minimize tampering.

Additional measures, such as the provision of crutches for injuries on feet, may be warranted.

Immunization

Effective tetanus prophylaxis is always of high priority when skin or mucosa has been violated traumatically.

If a child has had basic immunization and it has not been more than 5 years since the last booster, there is no need for a booster with the injury unless it is suspected to be heavily contaminated with *Clostridium*.

When there is doubt concerning the child's basic immunization status, he or she should be assumed to be nonimmunized and in need of human antitetanus globulin as well as initiation of active tetanus immunization. Arrangements must be made to ensure that the course of needles will be completed.

A baby seen for a laceration who has only had a first tetanus toxoid injection is considered nonimmunized. The baby who has had two injections of the basic course may be considered immunized and will need a booster only if 5 years have elapsed since the last dose.

Discharge Instructions, Suture Removal, and Arranging Follow-up

There can be no set policy that is appropriate for every instance. The important thing is for the physician to *think* and then to arrange whatever follow-up method is best for the patient.

If there is a high risk of infection, the child should be seen again in 2 or 3 days, long before suture removal time. In many institutions it is customary to refer a child back to the regular physician for suture removal. However, if their removal will be particularly difficult, it may be preferable to return the child to the hospital (i.e., the surgical clinic), where all facilities are available, including nurses who have experience in holding children for procedures. This applies especially to those areas on the body for which effective restraint is difficult, such as the chin or fingers, when very small stitches have been inserted, or if struggles can be anticipated.

With struggling, uncooperative children, it is often best to leave stitches in a day or so longer than one would in a comparable laceration in an adult. The procedure of suture removal is occasionally as physically vigorous an exercise as the laceration repair was, and one extra day of healing may decrease the risk of the cut being pulled open during the procedure. Furthermore, some children move around a great deal, rub and scratch themselves when they sleep, and may pull open cuts from which the suture material has just been removed. One extra day of healing decreases this risk remarkably. Facial sutures may be left in place for 6 days, as opposed to the 4 or 5 days usually selected for adults. Sutures should be left in scalps and shoulders for a week or so; those over the extensor surface of joints may need 10 or 12 days before removal is safe.

On the other hand, several absorbable subcuticular stitches to take tension off the skin closure may permit earlier suture removal and, hence, lessen the residual stitch marks. Adhesive strips applied after suture removal may serve the same purpose if one can ensure that they stay in place for a few days.

When a laceration lies over a joint, the movement of that joint may have to be restricted for a further few days after suture removal. For this reason a bulky bandage may be as important after the stitches come out of a knee laceration as it was before suture removal.

Written discharge instructions are of the utmost importance. Indeed, the record of the instructions given is important for the physician's legal protection.

Make sure parents know what to expect and what to look for. Explain carefully what to do in all eventualities and what their follow-up instructions are. Make sure they know how to make any needed appointments.

Medical Record

Before beginning the repair make sure a valid consent for treatment has been signed and is on the chart. If a valid consent is not available, consideration must be given to a telephone consent or to proceeding without parental consent if that is clinically necessary. When a valid parental consent cannot be obtained, some jurisdictions will accept consent from an intelligent, competent patient, even though he or she may be underage, provided the patient is able to understand the possible complications and outcomes when this is discussed (common law). Sometimes one needs to delay the treatment of a minor laceration if parental consent is expected to be available in an hour or so. Administrative or legal advice is desirable in difficult situations of this nature, and one should not hesitate to hold up treatment briefly for nonemergency situations to obtain this advice. The accuracy and completeness of the medical record become of great importance when complications arise as a result of injury, when subsequent illness or accident makes knowledge of this visit valuable, or when legal action is taken.

There are seven basic areas that should be covered on the chart:
1. History should be recorded. How did it happen?
2. The laceration should be described. A sketch is a good method.
3. There must be clear indication that the physician has thought about complications or associated injuries. For scalp lacerations there should be comment on the risk of cerebral concussion, and reference to the neurologic status of the patient and need for skull radiographs. For a cut on the palm, assessment of tendon and nerve function must be recorded. When a chin is cut in a fall, the chart must indicate that the physician has looked for signs of a fracture of the mandible, particularly in the region of the subcondylar neck on the side opposite to the laceration. If the lesion is caused by a vehicular accident, the general survey looking for other injuries should be described.
4. Pre-existing or associated medical conditions need to be mentioned. Allergies, particularly to drugs, should be noted as well as what measures are usually required to deal with them. Bleeding tendencies and conditions affecting resistance to infection are also important. Cardiac anomalies may warrant prophylactic antibiotic therapy if there is a risk of endocarditis. Other conditions may affect a child's ability to walk with crutches or a joint's ability to tolerate a period of immobilization.
5. Treatment should be described. What drug was used for local anesthesia? What suture material? A sketch showing the technique of closure is again often the best way to describe it. If the dressing is other than a Band-Aid or simple gauze and tape, it should be described.

6. The state of the child's immunizations should be on the chart as well as a note of any booster administered.

7. The follow-up advice and any recommendations given to parents must be recorded. To have recorded that instructions such as "the child must be seen here at once if there is any redness or swelling" or "report immediately any headaches, drowsiness, or vomiting" were transmitted to the parents is very reassuring when a case is investigated after the fact. This type of entry on the chart is for the benefit of both the patient and the physician. Finally, a note on the chart should indicate who will be seeing the child with a laceration in follow-up and when that is to be. *There must always be a physician's signature.*

Each patient deserves top-quality care. If the physician doubts his or her ability to provide it, he or she should request help. When a physician proceeds without making any attempt to learn from others, it is unfair to parents and child. Even if one has treated many lacerations and has read this or other guides, it is still very helpful to have somebody demonstrate some of the tricks in handling the difficult young child with a laceration before treating one for the first time.

Head and Neck

The Face

Trauma

A facial fracture should be suspected and sought with trauma around the eyes, to the cheek eminences, to the nose, or around the mouth or chin. When examining for a facial fracture, palpate orbital margins, the zygomata, and the nose for deformity or tenderness; visualize the nasal septum and both nasal airways; and check for dental tenderness, stability, and accuracy of occlusion. Look for mandibular tenderness, deformity, and function and particularly make sure the mandible remains central on opening widely. With a chin laceration, check particularly for a fracture of the subcondylar neck of the mandible on the side opposite to the laceration.

Special radiographs are available (e.g., Panorex). However, routine facial views plus stereo-Waters' views are usually adequate in the emergency situation. On these films, in addition to looking for fractures, check for air in bony spaces that do not normally contain air (e.g., the orbit or the anterior cranial fossa).

Blowout Fracture of the Orbit

A blowout fracture of the orbit should be suspected and looked for whenever there has been trauma to or around the eye. In a blowout fracture, direct trauma to the eye produces anteroposterior compression of the globe. This compression causes the globe to expand in the superior-inferior direction and applies pressure to the paper-thin orbital floor, which cracks very easily.

Diplopia on looking up and limitation of upward gaze of the involved eye are characteristic of a blowout fracture. These symptoms may be produced by entrapment of the inferior ocular muscles, particularly the inferior rectus, in the fracture line or possibly by restriction of inferior rectus function by the hemorrhage and reaction about the fracture. On radiograph clouding of the antrum because of bleeding from the fracture supports the diagnosis.

Nasal Trauma

Nasal trauma is common. Although the nose should be carefully palpated and the septum examined, general inspection of the nose gives the most useful information. Nasal fracture with deviation may be obvious. However, swelling may be so marked as to obscure deviation. When it is unclear, re-examination after 4 or 5 days, when the swelling has largely subsided, may reveal deviation. Further delay in reduction is undesirable because after the fifth or sixth day fractures begin to unite and manipulation becomes increasingly difficult. After the initial trauma, the parents should be asked to observe if the nose appears normal. If the nose looks crooked now, parents will know if it looked crooked before. Nasal radiographs are difficult to interpret and of relative usefulness only.

A septal hematoma should be looked for also. A hematoma can appear anytime in the first 48 hours after trauma. Therefore, even if the septum looks normal initially, the patient should be seen again within 2 or 3 days if the blow was significant and should definitely be reviewed at once if any obstruction to the nasal airway develops. An untreated septal hematoma can become infected, and the subsequent septal abscess may result in a septal perforation, the prevention of which hinges on early detection and prompt drainage of the initial traumatic septal hematoma.

Major Maxillary Fractures

Major maxillary fractures, usually with depression or instability of the maxilla, can result in major intraoral bleeding and shock. Such cases need prompt referral after resuscitative measures have been taken. As an interim measure, postnasal packing may offer some control of the hemorrhage.

Facial Lacerations

Facial lacerations are managed under the same principles of treatment that apply elsewhere, with increased concern about the cosmetic outcome being the chief practical difference. Lacerations of the lips are common in the 1- to 3-year-old child, who falls frequently. These need careful apposition with anatomic realignment of the vermilion border. Local anesthetic infiltration of the lips is easy and very effective because of the loose nature of the labial tissue. Sutures in the cutaneous portion of the lip should be nonabsorbable, whereas a rapidly absorbed catgut material is most suitable for the mucous membrane.

Lacerations of the Tongue

Lacerations of the tongue heal well in most instances without repair but will need to be sutured if there is persistent bleeding, if a large food pocket develops, or if a flap is produced that the child persists in chewing on or manipulating. Small lesions can be repaired with one or two simple sutures with the help of full restraints and a mouth gag. Efforts may be made to infiltrate the area with epinephrine containing local anesthesia, although the technical difficulties in administering the injection and in achieving adequate anesthesia persuade many to omit anesthesia for repairs requiring no more than one or two stitches. If more are needed, consideration should be given to repair under general anesthesia. All tongue lacerations that have been sutured should be followed carefully because, from time to time, hemorrhage within the tongue parenchyma can continue after the repair and cause such marked enlargement of the lingual bulk that the airway becomes partly obstructed.

Injuries to the External Ear

Injuries to the external ear are not common but require special consideration when they are seen. Following contusion injury to the pinna, subperichondrial bleeding can produce a hematoma, which may result in the classic cauliflower ear. The hematoma should be evacuated and the risk of recurrence minimized by the application of a pressure dressing.

Ear lacerations are fairly easily anesthetized and repaired using fine nonabsorbable sutures with careful apposition. Some lacerations of the cartilage can be easily sutured with fine absorbable material, although many will not need surgical referral. After repair, a pressure bandage around the head for a day or two is warranted to minimize bleeding and decrease the risk of hematoma formation.

Infection

Infection in the orbit is discussed in Chapter 12.

Boils, or other superficial infections of the face, are managed as they are elsewhere with the exception of those in the central third of the face, which drain to the cavernous venous sinus. Infections in this area require aggressive antibiotic therapy and strict avoidance of manipulation of the lesion lest this produce dissemination of infecting organisms into the cavernous system.

Cellulitis of the face in infancy is often due to *Haemophilus influenzae*, and aggressive broad-spectrum therapy is warranted. In such cases bacteremia is common, and there is risk of meningeal seeding.

Although the usual cause of acute parotitis is infection with the mumps virus, nonmumps parotitis also occurs from time to time and can be recurrent, whether caused by a stricture in the duct or partial obstruction from a small stone. For acute nonmumps parotitis not caused by a palpable or radiopaque stone, broad-spectrum antibiotic therapy, regular massage of the gland and duct forward toward the punctum of the duct, and frequent gum-chewing assist in the resolution of infection.

Epistaxis

The usual nosebleed is from the anterior septum and can be stopped by gentle "pinch" pressure for 10 minutes with the child sitting up. For a child with frequent nosebleeds, advice to the parents should include increasing the humidity in the home, application of sterile petrolatum (Vaseline) to the septum several times a day to minimize drying and crusting, and instructions on how to stop the bleeding with local pressure.

When simple measures fail to stop the episode, the application of 5% cocaine, with 1/10,000 epinephrine to achieve topical anesthesia, permits petrolatum gauze packing. (Some use oxidized cellulose [Oxycel].) Referral to an ear, nose, and throat specialist is necessary if the hemorrhage persists or if recurrences indicate the need for cauterization.

Lesions of the Eye

Trauma

For all trauma cases, careful assessment of visual acuity to the extent permitted by the age of the child and the presenting complaint is essential and must be recorded. This of the utmost importance, both medically and legally. Pain in the eye and visual deficiency following trauma imply potentially serious injury and must be treated seriously.

Subconjunctival Hematoma

When there is a localized collection of blood deep to the superficial conjunctiva, it remains bright red until it is absorbed because oxygen diffuses through the conjunctiva and keeps the hemoglobin oxygenated. Subconjunctival hematomas are usually due to trauma, although conjunctivitis sometimes causes one to appear. Rarely a subconjunctival hematoma heralds an underlying penetrating injury. In the absence of other lesions, the hematoma itself is unimportant.

Foreign Body

When a patient complains "there's something in my eye," the sensation is usually due to direct irritation of the corneal conjunctiva by a foreign body. Corneal abrasions or lesions of the lid margins may cause the same sensation, and occasionally it is a symptom of conjunctivitis.

The individual may be able to point to the site of the object. If the source of irritation is not readily visible, the upper and lower conjunctival fornices should be examined and the upper lid everted to permit better visualization of its inner surface. If a foreign body is noted, it should be lifted off with a moistened cotton swab. Topical anesthesia can be used to relieve discomfort, relax the patient, and facilitate examination and removal of the particle. Staining with a fluorescein strip helps when difficulty is encountered locating the object. If the foreign body is noted to be on the bulbar conjunctiva, it can usually be lifted off with the point of a fine needle after topical anesthesia is administered. If nothing is discovered and the sensation persists, referral is required.

Corneal Abrasion

Scratches or abrasions on the cornea arise from direct trauma or a previous foreign body. Erosions or scratches in the global conjunctiva are easily revealed by fluorescein staining. If there is no other lesion, a topical antibiotic ointment or drops, plus a patch for 24 hours, will permit complete healing. A follow-up referral to an ophthalmologist to confirm healing is warranted. Immediate referral is advised if neither abrasion nor foreign body is noted in the presence of persisting symptoms.

Lid Lacerations

Most lacerations are horizontally oriented, superficial, and readily repaired. However, if the laceration involves the lid margin or the medial canthus where the nasolacrimal duct is situated, referral for repair is indicated. Whenever the lid is traumatized, careful examination of the globe is important to rule out associated hyphema or other damage.

Hyphema

Blood in the anterior chamber is a frequent outcome of direct trauma. It is seen as a blurring of the red reflex on ophthalmoscopy, a general haziness, or layering in the lower quadrant if the child is sitting up. A hyphema may take a few hours to appear. Care should be taken to look for more serious associated eye injuries.

Hyphemas should all be referred for a complete ophthalmologic examination. Hospital admission is frequently warranted.

Potentially Serious Injuries

Possible perforation or laceration of the globe or an intraocular foreign body is often suspected from history. Sudden pain in the eye when hammering or striking a rock suggests a projected foreign body. Following direct trauma, photophobia, lid spasm, pain, and visual defect are ominous signs. Inspection may reveal a corneal laceration, prolapse of the iris, or softening or obvious shrinking down of the globe. All these require skilled care by a specialist. When there is marked blepharospasm, the lids should not be forced open. Both eyes should be covered with sterile dressings. The child should be kept supine and referred.

Chemical Burn

Acids or alkalis may corrode the conjunctiva and cause deeper damage if not quickly removed. The eye should be irrigated copiously with water or saline for 10 to 15 minutes. All particulate matter (e.g., lime) should be washed out. This may require eversion of the upper lid. When irrigation is complete the child should be referred to an ophthalmologist.

The Red Eye

Visible redness of the eyeball is due to vascular congestion, which may be conjunctival or ciliary.

Conjunctival Congestion

Congestion of the conjunctiva causes redness most intense in the conjunctival sac and on the conjunctival surface of the lids, with very little in the pericorneal area. This congestion is usually due to a *bacterial conjunctivitis*, which produces a mucopurulent discharge that is easily demonstrated and causes the lids to be stuck together when the child awakens from sleep. There is no pain, and vision remains normal.

Sulfacetamide sodium (10%) drops during the day are quite effective. The ointment form is better if there is inflammation of the lid margins. Although topical treatment is preferred, broad-spectrum antibiotics administered systemically are also effective. If the inflammation is severe or does not respond, if there is a membrane, or if the lids are inflamed, referral is indicated.

Ciliary Congestion

Ciliary congestion is caused by *acute keratitis, acute glaucoma* (rare in children), or *acute iridocyclitis* (inflammation of the anterior uvea). In these conditions, congestion is most intense near the cornea because of dilatation of the deeper radioscleral vessels. Emergency consultation is indicated.

Orbital Cellulitis

Infection in the tissues of the orbit, around the globe, is infrequent but potentially very serious. Orbital cellulitis affects all ages but is most common in infancy. Although an upper respiratory infection may precede it, an insect bite or a facial abrasion occasionally seems to provide the route of entry.

There is edema, redness, and tenderness of the eyelids. Proptosis is sometimes detectable, and there is usually restriction of ocular movement. Visual acuity and fundoscopic examination remain normal until late. There may be little systemic toxicity early on. However, if systemic toxicity progresses and is marked, this should suggest septic thrombosis of the cavernous sinus.

The most common organism is *Haemophilus influenzae*, although gram-positive organisms are possibilities. Blood cultures are usually positive, emphasizing the risk of blood-borne infection, such as septicemia and meningitis.

Oral ampicillin is effective early in the disease when there are no systemic manifestations. Otherwise admission for aggressive intravenous therapy is indicated. Ophthalmologic consultation is also warranted.

13

Inflammatory Masses

General Considerations

Inflamed masses in the neck may arise from cervical lymph nodes or from infected congenital cysts of some sort, such as midline dermoid cysts or thyroglossal duct cysts. The vast majority are of lymph node origin, and these are chiefly in the anterior cervical triangle. Neoplastic enlargement of cervical nodes is more likely to occur in the posterior triangle.

Midline Dermoid Cysts

The congenital midline dermoid cyst is often noted anteriorly just above the sternal notch. In this site, there is difficulty in establishing that the cyst is freely mobile and not connected deeply behind the sternum. Excision by the surgeon is usually easy, providing it does prove to be a midline dermoid cyst and not a thymic lesion (e.g., choristoma). When the cyst is infected, initial drainage to resolve the infection first is necessary and can be followed by elective excision after the inflammation has subsided. Other infrequent sites for this lesion are the thyroid or submental areas.

Thyroglossal Duct Cyst

An inflamed cystic mass in the midline over the thyroid area probably represents infection arising in a pre-existing thyroglossal duct cyst. Because complete thyroglossal remnant excision is very difficult in the presence of infection, prompt elective excision before it becomes infected is important. After infection has produced an abscess, however, the treatment is initial drainage and resolution of the infection, with subsequent total elective excision.

Cervical Adenitis and Abscess

Inflammation of lymph glands in the neck is very common. The glands most commonly involved are the deep cervical below the mandibular angle, although submental or submandibular adenitis is also seen. Nodes can be palpable in other areas, such as in the posterior triangle, postauricular area, and suboccipital area, but nodes in these sites rarely enlarge significantly from infection, and abscesses from them are rare.

Most acute cervical lymphadenitis is due to *Staphylococcus aureus* or *Streptococcus hemolyticus*. When the inflammatory reaction is particularly indolent, other causative agents should also be considered. Two possibilities are the atypical acid-fast mycobacteria, or chromogens, and the cat-scratch virus. With the latter, there will usually be a history of a cat-scratch within the previous few weeks.

Some systemic illnesses, such as infectious mononucleosis, cause generalized lymphadenitis most marked in the cervical area. Careful examination usually reveals nodes elsewhere.

The primary site of infection in most instances of cervical adenitis is obscure, although occasionally an infected lesion of the scalp can be found. The nasopharynx is a likely site of origin for some infections.

The mass will initially be firm and tender but nonfluctuant. Without antibiotics one can expect it to become soft and ready for drainage within a week or so. There are exceptions that take much longer, particularly if antibiotic therapy has been used.

For typical early cervical adenitis, a course of cloxacillin is usually worthwhile. One can expect streptococcal adenitis to respond readily. Staphylococcal adenitis will also respond but to a satisfactory degree only in the early stages before advanced suppuration has occurred. If there is not a good response within 8 to 10 days, the drugs should be stopped and fluctuation permitted to progress without further delay, unless there is marked systemic toxicity requiring systemic therapy. Stopping the drugs promptly and completely results in earlier maturation of the abscess.

Surgical drainage of a cervical abscess should be delayed until the skin overlying it is thinned out and the abscess visibly pointing. If the abscess is drained at this stage, disappearance of the mass will be rapid and complete healing of the wound will be prompt. If drainage is carried out too soon, the mass will still be thick-walled and will neither collapse down as satisfactorily nor heal as rapidly. Some physicians restart antibiotics after drainage in the hope of decreasing the risk of pyemia, although this benefit has not been statistically established.

From time to time a child is seen who has been treated for cervical adenitis for several weeks with different types of antibiotic and has had only limited response. In this situation, it is usually desirable to stop all antibiotics until fluctuation has progressed to a stage permitting surgical drainage.

14

Acute Torticollis

General Considerations

In acute torticollis, or acute wry neck, there are limitation of rotation and lateral flexion of the neck, pain due to muscle spasm, and visible postural deformity.

Spontaneous Torticollis

In spontaneous torticollis, there is no history of trauma, although there may be an intercurrent respiratory infection. The attack may seem to be precipitated by a trivial head movement, holding the head in one position for a long time, or a cold draft.

There is fixed torsion of the head and neck produced by muscle spasm, mainly of the trapezius and deeper muscles posteriorly, less so of the sternomastoid. The child is fearful of any movement and of the examination and usually supports the head with one or both hands. Rotation toward the painful side is particularly uncomfortable and is resisted.

Manual longitudinal traction (pulling on the head) with the patient supine for 10 minutes may give relief from the pain and spasm and may facilitate examination because it then permits neck movement for a brief interval. Tenderness is noted over the muscles posteriorly, not over spinal structures.

Good radiographs are difficult to obtain because of the rotatory deformity and rarely reveal anything of significance in the spontaneous variety of torticollis. Consequently, radiographs are not often warranted.

Treatment consists of the following:
1. *Analgesics.*
2. *Heat.*

3. *Muscle Relaxant.* This is of doubtful effectiveness, although the systemic calming effect of diazepam may be useful.
4. *Cervical ruff.* This is certainly not needed in very mild cases. However, when pain is moderate or severe, it may be useful and can facilitate sitting or standing up.
5. *Admission for traction.* When the discomfort is particularly severe or fails to respond, admission to the hospital for a period of halter traction may be required.

The response to treatment is usually rapid, and symptoms generally subside within 1 to 3 days.

Post-Traumatic Torticollis

Post-traumatic torticollis occurs after torsion or flexion stress to the neck, as may be encountered in wrestling or gymnastics. The clinical presentation is similar to that of the spontaneous variety.

Investigation is important in traumatic conditions. Radiographs to rule out facet overriding or fracture are necessary. Some attribute the picture to a rotatory subluxation of C1 on C2, although this is a very controversial condition and not all agree to its existence. If there is no abnormality on the plain films of the cervical spine, flexion-extension films may be warranted but should be done with neurosurgical supervision.

If skeletal abnormalities are demonstrated, referral is required. If no skeletal lesion is demonstrated, the treatment is similar to that for spontaneous torticollis and response should be rapid.

15

Foreign Bodies

General Considerations

The variety of objects that are inserted into the nose or ear is legion. These vary from pieces of sponge, beans, peas, popcorn, raisins, and erasers to the more exotic, such as lumps of rabbit excreta or gold keepers from expensive earrings. Although most foreign bodies are completely innocuous in themselves, their mechanical presence may be irritating to tissues and can result in inflammation. Biologic products may absorb water and swell in situ, resulting in obstruction of the passage, pressure on the adjacent tissue, and increased difficulty in removal.

Other objects are ingested and may introduce the risk of gastrointestinal perforation or obstruction. Ingestion of foreign bodies occurs in the young child or toddler who explores and learns by putting objects into the mouth or the older child who inadvertently swallows what he or she was holding in the mouth. Occasionally ingestion is intentional and may even indicate a psychiatric illness.

Of all the possible routes of entry into the body, aspiration has the most serious potential for complications. Possible inhalation of a foreign body must be considered when there are otherwise unexplained respiratory symptoms.

Although most instances of foreign body insertion occur in the toddler or preschooler, the older child or even teenager may inadvertently or absent-mindedly shove something in the ear. The swallowing of large numbers of foreign bodies such as nails or pieces of glass is frequently reported and may be a combination of a suicidal gesture and an attention-getting device.

Small insects sometimes crawl into the external ear canal and seek refuge against the drum, where removal becomes difficult. This can occur in any age group.

Foreign bodies are the chief cause of purulent vaginal discharge in the young child. These are discussed in Chapter 32.

All in all, the clinical manifestations of ingestion, aspiration, and insertion of foreign bodies are protean. When attempting to understand a vague or unexplained clinical picture, particularly in a young child, foreign body causation must always be considered.

The clinical manifestations of the presence of a foreign body depend on the anatomic site. History, however, is of its usual importance, and one point is of particular relevance. When a parent suspects a child has shoved into the nose or ear, has swallowed, or has choked on a foreign body, this should be considered as the number one possibility.

Foreign Bodies Up the Nose

Except for the child who arrives saying he or she shoved something up the nose, or the parent who claims to have seen the actual insertion, most intranasal foreign bodies are discovered when the physician looks into a nose being examined for persistent purulent, often foul-smelling, discharge.

With satisfactory lighting and restraint, removal with an ear loop, a small spoon, or long fine forceps is usually not difficult. In some instances insertion of a cotton pledget soaked in 2% cocaine will facilitate foreign body removal by providing both shrinkage of the edematous mucosa and topical anesthesia. Indeed, the object sometimes falls out as the pledget is removed. If the foreign body is too far up for easy extraction, or if it pushes ahead of the forceps and there is risk of it being aspirated, referral is warranted. Expulsion of the object can sometimes be achieved by blowing sharply into the child's mouth while the unaffected nostril is occluded.

Foreign Bodies In the Ear

Intra-aural foreign bodies rarely cause symptoms and may be discovered incidentally when a child is undergoing a routine examination. A child may be seen putting something in the ear, and when the physician is then consulted and looks into the canal, he or she may discover that the offending object is only one of many previously inserted.

Removal is usually accomplished simply using an ear loop. For objects that seem stuck or are firmly against the drum, referral to an ear, nose, and throat specialist is prudent.

Some objects are best and most safely removed by syringing. Insects deep in the canal may float up on saline or oil, which, for comfort, should be at body temperature.

Ingested Foreign Bodies

Children somehow manage to swallow almost anything that can pass through the pharynx. The child will usually indicate when the object is stuck in the pharynx or esophagus and may point to its exact location. A foreign body lodged in the esophagus will usually cause drooling or vomiting because of obstruction and may even induce dyspnea because of local pressure on the adjacent trachea. When parents volunteer that their child choked, turned blue, gagged, and then was all right, ingestion or aspiration of a foreign body is the first possibility to be considered.

Fortunately most ingested foreign bodies cause no trouble and pass through the intestinal tract uneventfully. In such cases, radiographs serve several purposes. It is important to establish that the object was, indeed, ingested and not aspirated, so demonstrating its presence in the stomach has value even though it only rarely leads to any intervention. Proving the nature of the foreign body and demonstrating that it should be completely innocuous is reassuring. When a parent suspects a child has swallowed a metallic object, demonstrating on radiograph that there is no radiopaque foreign body to be found eliminates a great deal of concern and the need for follow-up.

Any radiographic study designed to look for an ingested or aspirated foreign body should include the body from incisors to anus. Too often an elusive foreign body is belatedly discovered residing in the nasopharynx, which was not included on the initial chest or abdominal film.

When a radiopaque foreign body has been demonstrated in the stomach, two situations warrant careful follow-up. If the object is potentially dangerous, as might be the case with a long straight pin or an open safety pin, or if its size suggests the risk of its becoming firmly lodged in the tract somewhere, periodic follow-up and radiographic study to establish progress are warranted. In an attempt to minimize radiation, it is often useful to direct parents to continue to examine the child's stools, using a tongue depressor or similar tool until the object has been expelled.

Any object shown to be lodged in the esophagus should be referred for consideration of endoscopic removal.

Although most ingested foreign bodies are radiopaque, some are not, and this possibility must be entertained when the clinical picture suggests the presence of a foreign body that cannot be demonstrated on radiograph.

Aspirated Foreign Bodies

Aspiration of a foreign body is suggested by an episode of coughing, choking, or gagging, especially in the presence of one of the objects that is notorious for aspiration. Such objects are peanuts, pieces of raw carrots or other vegetables, fragments of small toys, and heads from various grains (e.g., flax or rye). The peanut has for decades been the most common foreign body to be aspirated. Peanuts should not be available to toddlers until they reach age 4 or 5, when they have developed their full molar dentition and can properly grind such objects to a pulp.

The clinical picture of an aspirated foreign body frequently simulates asthma, particularly in a child not known to be asthmatic. Indeed, for any first attack of asthma, the presence of a foreign body should be considered. Chronic or recurring cough or repeated chest "infections" should be examined from the point of view of a foreign body. Rarely an audible click is produced by a foreign body moving freely in the trachea.

Radiographic study may be completely normal, or it may show overinflation or collapse. Inspiratory and expiratory films are frequently of particular value. The customary finding is an expiration film showing the lung or lobe involved to remain inflated while the rest of the lung tissue deflates well.

When history, examination, or radiograph suggests foreign body aspiration, referral for consideration of bronchoscopy is indicated. The late complications of untreated foreign body aspiration (lung abscess, bronchiectasis) are sufficiently serious that endoscopy is indicated on reasonable suspicion only of aspiration. Many centers accept three or four negative bronchoscopies for every positive one, realizing that the damage done when an inhaled foreign body is missed is far greater than the risk from a negative bronchoscopy.

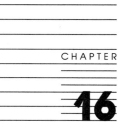
Acute Dental Conditions

Trauma

Chipped, fractured, or avulsed teeth are common in contact sports, playground accidents, and automobile accidents. Avulsions are usually seen in young adolescents, whereas chipped or fractured teeth occur most often in teenagers. Intrusions are common with deciduous teeth.

Teeth with small pieces fractured off the incisal edge or a corner missing may need only grinding or smoothing with sandpaper. This can be performed on a nonurgent basis by the family dentist. If dentin is visible in the surface defect, prompt referral to a dentist may be necessary because dentin is a vital and sensitive tissue and requires protection from the oral environment. The dentist will customarily cover the exposed dentin with a calcium hydroxide preparation.

More severe fractures may involve a large portion of the crown. If pulp is freshly exposed, it will be reddish in color. Exposed pulp is black if long-standing. Urgent dental care is needed if pulp has been exposed to save the tooth, control pain, and avoid infection. Fractures crossing the root are visible only on radiographs and require immediate dental referral when recognized.

The tooth most commonly avulsed is one of the permanent upper incisors. Such a tooth, although itself rendered nonvital, is the best form of prosthesis available from the point of view of aesthetics and space maintenance. Successful replantation hinges on the presence of surviving periodontal cells on the external surface of the root; the sooner the tooth is replanted following avulsion, the more likely will there be any surviving cells. A delay of 2 hours from avulsion is the maximum for satisfactory replantation. Cell survival is favored by storage of the tooth in a suitable medium. The tooth should be kept in cold, fresh milk or cold saline. It should not be kept ''on ice'' because freezing will render any remaining cells nonvital. It is probably best not to keep the avulsed tooth in the child's mouth as is so often recommended because of the risk of swallowing or aspiration. During manipulation, the tooth should be held by the crown so as not to damage the precious cell rests on the root surface that are so important in the success of the procedure. If the injury is very fresh, the tooth can usually be immediately replaced on site. The child should then be referred to his or her dentist for fixation of the tooth. If a clot has formed, it will need to be washed out under local anesthesia by a gentle stream of saline and will require dental attention.

Primary teeth are *never* replanted.

When a tooth is missing after facial trauma and cannot be found, a radiograph to include the area from mouth to diaphragm is required lest it be lodged somewhere in the mouth or pharynx or even in the lung. An abdominal film will show it if it has been ingested, although no harm is likely to come from a swallowed tooth.

Deciduous incisors are frequently injured because of every toddler's tendency to fall several times each day. A baby incisor tends to shift en masse rather than chip or fracture, and the common result is bodily luxation or intrusion. Such teeth can be moved lingually, labially, or even driven up out of sight, totally embedded within the gum. Dental advice is clearly needed with these conditions, although no harm will come from a few hours' delay unless the tooth is sufficiently loose that it may come free and be aspirated. When a deciduous incisor has been traumatically shifted in any direction, the separation of its apical attachment is likely to produce a small hematoma, which in turn runs a high risk of becoming infected. An apical infection of a deciduous incisor jeopardizes the permanent tooth bud adjacent to it. Consequently, prevention by extraction of the intruded incisor when initially seen or soon after is frequently indicated.

Toothache

Many toothaches are caused by the irritation of pulp contents by the proximity of the pulp to the surface of the tooth, which is the result of dental caries. Others arise when the pulpal irritation is long-standing and infection has been introduced and has resulted in pulpal necrosis. This causes an apical abscess. Differentiation of pulpal irritation from established abscess is important in assessing the degree of urgency with which dental advice is needed.

The pain originating within a cavity comes in sharp stabs, usually produced by cold liquids or breathing in cold air by mouth. The cavity is usually visible; in fact, such a complaint often occurs in a mouth in which the teeth are obviously carious. One does not see with a cavity the gingival inflammation characteristic of an abscess.

Symptomatic relief can be obtained in most instances by the application into the cavity of a small pledget of cotton batten soaked in eugonol. This is, of course, a temporary measure, and more permanent dental care is required in due course.

If previously experienced, the pain of a subsequent dental abscess is likely to be identified correctly by the patient. Consequently, a patient who thinks he or she has an abscess probably does. The pain of an abscess is usually throbbing and worsens on contact with warm water. Conversely, it may be relieved completely by holding cold water in the mouth. Tapping the offending tooth with a tongue depressor or a spoon causes marked pain, and pressure on the tooth in chewing is very painful. The patient may volunteer that the tooth feels as if it protrudes farther than normal. Examination of the gum over the root of an abscessed tooth reveals edema, redness, glossy appearance, and marked tenderness. Some apical abscesses will even drain externally through the labial surface of the mucosa (gumboil).

An apical abscess requires drainage, either by dental extraction or by a root canal procedure. However, because most dentists prefer to delay drainage to permit 12 to 18 hours of antibiotic coverage, dental attention at the end of that period is usually satisfactory. Rarely is the pain severe enough to require immediate drainage.

Head Injuries

General Considerations

Head injuries of various degrees of severity are very common in the pediatric age group, partly because the head is relatively large and heavy in proportion to body size. Coordination that is as yet undeveloped and vigorous activities by children who display little caution and possess no sense of risk also contribute. Head injuries, either associated with other injuries or alone, are a major cause of death and permanent disability in the young. Fortunately, many mild head injuries have no untoward sequelae with long-term effect.

Causes

In young infants, falls from dressing tables, from parent's arms, or from strollers or carriages are frequent causes of head injures. Injuries also occur in babies when moving about in walkers or other baby appliances. Toddlers injure heads often by falling or running into furniture. An unrestrained infant may be thrown about within a vehicle involved in a road accident or may be expelled from the vehicle.

Older preschoolers fall from playground equipment (especially slides) or run into the path of vehicles. They may also fall from apartment balconies or upper-floor windows. Vehicle-pedestrian accidents are common in children aged 3 or 4 and usually cause multiple injuries with great mortality and long-term morbidity.

Schoolchildren fall from bicycles, trees, or windows and at that age are beginning to play contact sports, in which minor head injuries are common. Older children are injured in car-bicycle accidents, contact sports, incidents involving toboggans, skateboards, and so forth.

Abuse

Abuse must be kept in mind as a possible cause of cerebral injury with or without skull fracture. The history of every accident must be examined carefully to avoid missing abuse. For example, the distance of the "fall" is important. A baby does not sustain a parietal skull fracture falling less than 2 feet from the bed to a broadloom rug. Several skull fracture lines visible on the radiograph of a small baby are highly suspicious of abuse, unless there is an obvious explanation. Retinal hemorrhages suggest a subdural hematoma and are frequently noted in babies who have sustained shaking.

Skull Fractures

Skull fractures are common. The presence of a scalp contusion or hematoma is an important clue to an underlying fracture. A fracture of the vault is almost always associated with some external evidence of trauma. This is particularly true in infancy, when an overlying cephalhematoma, which may take some days to appear, should alert one to the fracture. Traumatic widening of a suture (traumatic diastasis or a diastatic fracture) has the same significance as a fracture line. In children there is much less correlation between a parietal fracture and a developing extradural hematoma than in adults. Fortunately, nondepressed fractures require no definitive treatment, provided there is no overlying laceration converting the fracture to an open one. The finding of a simple linear fracture of the vault is of relatively little significance from the medical point of view, and care must be taken not to exaggerate its importance.

Open fractures require formal operative debridement and closure. Depressed fractures are uncommon but important to recognize because surgical elevation is necessary in the majority. Such a depression is usually caused by a localized blow from a blunt object, such as a golf club, hammer, or thrown rock, and it is striking how often there is no indication of associated cerebral injury.

The distance of the fall and the type of landing surface, the history of a blow from a blunt object, or a large cephalhematoma should alert one to situations in which fractures are likely.

Clinical Features

Detailed history is all-important and may be the chief indicator of the severity of trauma.

Drowsiness, vomiting, and headache all suggest the postconcussion syndrome and should gradually subside in hours or a day or so.

However, because these symptoms can also be produced by increased intracranial pressure, the timing and sequence of their occurrence must be carefully analyzed. Consciousness that fails to improve rapidly after seemingly minor trauma or that deteriorates after initially improving is suggestive of increasing space occupation by a clot. Similarly, a severe headache beginning 8 to 12 hours following trauma may be the first indication of a developing clot.

A complete general physical examination is required. The patient must be undressed even if the head injury seems minor because associated injuries may remain undiscovered unless sought.

Blood in the middle ear indicates fracture of the petrous temporal bone. If there is bleeding from the ear canal and it is not clear whether the blood is coming from a laceration of the canal or from the middle ear through a tympanic rupture, the differentiation can often be made through a simple hearing test. Marked deafness suggests that a basal fracture with hematotympanum is more likely to be the source of the blood than a laceration of the external canal.

Cerebrospinal fluid rhinorrhea is a sign of a cribriform plate fracture. However, allergic rhinitis may be very similar in presentation to cerebrospinal fluid rhinorrhea, and differentiation is not always simple. The nasal discharge of allergy usually subsides when the child sleeps; cerebrospinal fluid drainage continues. A brow-up lateral radiograph revealing an anterior pneumocranium establishes the presence of a basal fracture, permitting the entrance of outside air and its organisms. Although small amounts of air in the anterior cranial fossa are readily missed on plain films, a computed tomographic (CT) scan will demonstrate even the tiniest collection and should be requested if there is any concern about cerebrospinal fluid rhinorrhea in a child whose radiograph seems normal.

Ecchymosis of the upper eyelids, sharply restricted superiorly to the supraorbital margin ("raccoon eyes"), suggests an anterior fossa basal fracture with bleeding first into the orbit and then outward into the lid. This diagnosis is most easily made when the external contusion is not close to the eyes. These fractures are often not demonstrated on routine radiography, so the diagnosis may be on clinical grounds only. If there are bilateral raccoon eyes, one should watch for cerebrospinal fluid rhinorrhea because the basal fracture may extend from one orbital roof to the other, crossing the cribriform plate en route.

A neurologic examination, checking specifically for cranial nerves, the motor system, the sensory system, and, if possible, cerebellar function, is essential and must be recorded. The examination should be as early after the incident as possible so that trends can be assessed. A facial nerve palsy immediately after head trauma means the nerve was damaged, probably irreparably, by the injury and may have been trapped or divided in a fracture. If the palsy is delayed for some hours, it suggests gradual compression by hemorrhage in the stylomastoid foramen; surgical decompression might be warranted. Other delayed neurologic deficits may be the first indication of a space-occupying clot within the skull.

An essential part of the neurologic examination of a patient with a head injury is the assessment, measurement, and recording of the

Table 17–1. Glasgow Coma Scale with Pediatric Modifications

EYE OPENING			BEST MOTOR RESPONSE			BEST VERBAL RESPONSE		
SCORE	0–12 mo	over 12 mo	SCORE	0–12 mo	over 12 mo	SCORE	0–23 mo	2–5 yr	over 5 yr
4	Spontaneously	Spontaneously	6	Normal	Obeys	5	Smiles, coos, cries appropriately	Appropriate words, phrases	Oriented, converses
3	To shout	To verbal command	5	Localizes pain	Localizes pain	4	Cries appropriately	Inappropriate words	Disoriented, converses
2	To pain	To pain	4	Flexion withdrawal	Flexion withdrawal	3	Inappropriate cries, screams	Cries, screams	Inappropriate words
1	No response	No response	3	Decorticate flexion	Decorticate flexion	2	Grunts	Grunts	Sounds not comprehensible
			2	Decerebrate extension	Decerebrate extension	1	No response	No response	No response
			1	No response	No response				

level of consciousness. Vague descriptive terms have been used to describe responses of the patient to various stimuli in the hope of portraying the level of consciousness. Much of the inherent inaccuracy has been eliminated by the adoption of the Glasgow Coma Scale, which permits numerical recording of three specific modalities of response to stimuli. This method permits different observers at different times to do the same examination and duplicate the results and, consequently, allows for much more effective following of the course of a patient's consciousness. Changes can now be recorded on paper in a simple numeric form (Table 17–1).

The 18-month-old infant whose eyes open to verbal command, who withdraws the hand or foot in response to pain, and who cries appropriately in response to discomfort has a score of $3+5+4=12$. Whenever the infant's consciousness is assessed, this should be recorded and graphed.

Assessment of the other vital signs is equally important in evaluating trauma victims, particularly those with head injuries. Pulse and blood pressure readings help in determining circulatory status and the possibility of hypovolemic shock. The autonomic system of the child is able to maintain circulation remarkably well even after significant blood loss. However, pallor and cold, clammy skin are seen early on and, when marked, may signify a hemorrhage of as much as one-fourth of normal blood volume even with normal pulse and blood pressure. When the signs of inadequate peripheral perfusion, along with hypotension and tachycardia, signal the presence of shock in a child with a head injury, one must look elsewhere for the source of hemorrhage. It is as true in children as it is in adults that head injuries do not cause shock. In these patients, it is a ruptured spleen or liver, a hemothorax, or a massive retroperitoneal hemorrhage from a fractured pelvis that causes hypovolemic shock. Only in the terminal stages of a severe brain injury will one see hypotension develop as a result of the head injury per se.

Skull Radiographs

Of all bumped heads, very few need to undergo radiography. However, depression of consciousness, neurologic deficit, or a large cephalhematoma warrants a routine skull series. Medicolegal situations are often stated to be indications for radiographic study. In these instances, careful medical assessment is far more important than the radiographs, and when there are no medical reasons to obtain radiographs, it is rare for legal reasons to justify obtaining them.

The importance of finding a linear skull fracture line on the radiograph and the degree to which this finding is permitted to influence management of the patient have been vastly exaggerated. The simple linear skull fracture causes more parental concern than it warrants and requires no treatment when it is detected. For practical purposes, there is a very little benefit in obtaining plain skull films unless a depressed fracture is suspected. In addition, many experts now believe clinical signs of a basal fracture are indications for a CT scan and that plain films are unnecessary.

The finding of a fracture crossing the middle meningeal groove does not have the ominous significance in the child that it does in the adult, in whom careful surveillance for an extradural hematoma would be warranted. There is little correlation in children between the presence of a fracture and the risk of a clot developing. Nor does absence of a fracture decrease the risk of an extradural hematoma. In children, the majority of extradural hematomas occur without fractures.

Many believe that the ideal form of radiographic investigation for head injuries arriving in the emergency department is to proceed directly to CT scan. This will probably be the routine in centers in which the facilities are available and may well be a more economical form of management.

Convulsions Following Trauma

From time to time a child will undergo a generalized convulsion within minutes of a mild head injury with no apparent sequelae. Such convulsions are not believed to be of major significance, and there is very questionable indication for continuing anticonvulsant therapy. This is in contrast to the convulsion occurring many days to weeks after the injury, at which time persisting cortical abnormality, such as an area of scarring, is more likely to be responsible.

Head Injury Routine

When there has been unconsciousness, however brief, a demonstrated skull fracture; or postconcussive symptoms that are particularly severe or persist for more than a few hours, it is traditional in most centers to admit the child for an arbitrary 1 to 2 days for observation. The rationale for this decision, although sometimes difficult to justify, is that when the trauma has been severe enough to result in marked symptoms or a fracture, one can infer an increased risk of a posttraumatic hemorrhage, which would be best diagnosed and treated in an already hospitalized patient. This is the basis for routine "head injury observation" orders, which list the specific vital signs to be given particular importance. How strictly these indications for admission are followed varies greatly from center to center. Sometime in the future the results of a routine computed tomographic scan on all such injured heads may be a much more useful criterion in deciding about admission and may, by avoiding many admissions, be a more economical way to make the decision.

When a patient is admitted for observation subsequent to a mild head injury, the basic indicators in the head injury routine that are followed are (1) level of consciousness, (2) pupils, (3) blood pressure, (4) pulse, and (5) respiration. Changes in these indicators produce the classic clinical picture of increased intracranial pressure resulting from an extradural clot over a cerebral hemisphere. Theoretically, there is a sequence in these alterations that should occur with this lesion, an understanding of which facilitates following the patient, although clinical examples of extradural hematomas do not very often follow exactly the textbook picture described herein.

The earliest change one should watch for is depression of consciousness caused by the effect of the early increase in pressure on the reticular activating substance. As pressure increases and is transmitted inferiorly through the hemisphere, the hippocampal gyrus is forced down around the free edge of the tentorium, pushing the ipsilateral oculomotor nerve ahead of it. This stretches the nerve and suppresses the pupillary constrictor function subserved by the parasympathetic fibers running with it, letting sympathetic dilator function predominate. The result is a gradually dilating pupil that is progressively less responsive to light and eventually becomes fixed and fully dilated. As time passes and near lethal pressure develops, the opposite pupil follows the same sequence. When both pupils are fully dilated and fixed, the child is not likely to survive, whatever the treatment.

As pupillary changes are becoming apparent, the pressure is also being felt in the midbrain and brain stem, where the resulting ischemic hypoxia causes the circulatory regulating center to respond by producing an increase in blood pressure. This hypertension, in turn, results in bradycardia, again through the circulatory regulating centers. Hypertension is essential for brain survival when there is increased pressure within the skull, and there must be no attempt to bring down what may be alarming hypertension until the pressure within the skull has been relieved.

As these changes progress, increased intracranial pressure ultimately affects the respiratory center, resulting in respiratory depression or Cheynes-Stokes respiration. When an extradural hematoma has caused all these physiologic changes to the point of respiratory depression, one can expect treatment to be ineffectual.

Occasionally the sequence of events with an extradural hematoma is atypical and does not follow the classic picture described. Rarely this is due to an atypical site for the clot. For example, a posterior fossa extradural hematoma is located below the tentorium and does not put pressure on the third cranial nerve, and there may be no pupillary signs until consciousness and other vital processes are markedly compromised.

The charting of a head injury routine is of the utmost importance. The level of consciousness should be described in words and given a Glasgow Coma Scale score. This and the other vital parameters should be graphed to provide an instantaneous picture of trends in the patient's condition.

Management

The basic management for mild head injuries consists of surveillance to detect developing complications when and where they can be most effectively treated. For more severe head injuries associated with un-

consciousness, referral and admission for more aggressive investigation and intensive care modalities are required. The percentage of
injured heads that require surgery is small.

The first and most important modality of treatment needed in significant head injuries, and the one least well provided but with the
greatest potential of saving lives, is proper airway and respiratory care.
Intubation and positive pressure ventilation, and in many cases hyperventilation, are essential in managing the moderate to severe brain contusion by controlling cerebral edema as well as maintaining oxygena-
tion of peripheral tissues. In children, delay in initiating these measures is the most common error in the early management of head injuries, and avoiding delay cannot be overemphasized.

Discharge Instructions

In the management of head injuries, proper discharge instructions for
those who are going home are as important for the safety of the patient as is the decision to admit for those who do not go home. Delayed
intracranial bleeding following trauma is so unpredictable that for the
child who is seen for a mild head injury and sent home, discharge instructions must focus on seeking help promptly if any indications of
intracranial bleeding are encountered. Any severe or increasing
headache, persistent vomiting, or, most importantly, increased drowsiness or difficulty in rousing should prompt immediate contact with
medical help. Parents must be told clearly whom to telephone or where
to go should any of the warning signs occur.

The Abdomen

18

Acute Abdominal Pain

General Considerations

Approach to Diagnosis

Acute abdominal pain is not only common as a presenting complaint in the pediatric age group, but also must always be considered as potentially serious. Although the majority of infants and children who present with abdominal pain do not have acute surgical conditions, a sufficient number do to make it necessary that acute surgical disease be sought in all. Furthermore, in the child who does not already have a surgical scar on the abdomen and in whom ovarian disease and trauma can be ruled out, the acute abdominal condition encountered that requires emergency surgery is, with rare exceptions, acute appendicitis. Consequently, until this diagnosis can with confidence be eliminated, any child being assessed because of acute abdominal pain must be evaluated as one who may harbor acute appendicitis. A comparable situation holds for infancy (neonates excluded), when intussusception is almost the only acute condition ever to require emergency laparotomy.

To be able to say to oneself when about to assess the 9-month-old infant with abdominal pain, "my main job here is to make sure this baby doesn't have an intussusception," or when preparing to evaluate the 5-year-old with abdominal pain and vomiting, "above all else I need to find out if this child has acute appendicitis," has great practical value when that infant is crying constantly or that 5-year-old is obviously going to be uncooperative and difficult to examine.

Intussusception and appendicitis are the two acute abdominal surgical diseases of which the misdiagnoses plague every emergency department that receives infants and children. Indeed, were we able to eliminate all instances of delayed or missed diagnoses of intussusception or appendicitis, we would be removing virtually all major diagnostic mistakes in the area of acute abdominal disease in the pediatric age group.

History and Physical Examination

The importance of an accurate and complete history in reaching a proper diagnosis is never more evident than it is in acute pediatric situations. However, children frequently have a variety of caregivers during any given week. Hence, the accuracy of historical information delivered by one parent may be highly suspect when it relates to a period during which the child was in the care of the other parent or a babysitter. Furthermore, the characteristics of a symptom such as pain, information that is sometimes of crucial importance in one's attempt to reach an accurate diagnosis, and that is normally obtained directly from the patient, are not available from the 6-month-old infant or the 1-year-old. These are all roadblocks to complete history-taking that are almost routine in pediatric practice. On the other hand, to be able to concentrate on one disease makes it easier to select the key questions and omit those that are not crucial.

When attempting to evaluate abdominal pain in the pediatric age group, one will encounter many delightful children who are completely cooperative and easy to examine. On the other hand, some children, more often the younger ones, are unduly frightened and quite unable to cooperate. Others seem to infer from their parent's obvious anxiety that they also should panic. The occasional child may be so spoiled and ill-behaved that one cannot envisage ever establishing sufficient rapport to carry out a satisfactory examination. Proper abdominal examination requires a degree of muscular relaxation that is probably unobtainable in a child who refuses to let go of his or her mother's neck. These situations occur regularly in pediatric emergency practice and clearly compromise diagnostic accuracy. As a result, one must make use of special techniques, tricks, and subterfuges to obtain rapport or, if rapport cannot be achieved, at least to fool the child into thinking he or she is not being examined.

Abdominal pain is often caused by lesions located outside the usually accepted boundaries of the abdomen itself. Pneumonia is probably the most common of these. Because testicular torsion or incarcerated inguinal hernia can also produce lower abdominal pain, it is important to inspect the external genitalia during examination.

The Record

The need for careful recording of essential information on the emergency chart is never greater than it is for the child with acute abdominal pain, particularly when that child is thought not to have a surgical condition and is being discharged. Within the account of the examination, emphasis must be placed on a description of the efforts taken to demonstrate peritoneal irritation. The chart should not just say "no peritoneal irritation." It must read "child could jump up and down without pain," "child willing to run up corridor without discomfort," or "no pain on vigorous shaking of pelvis." When a child is seen on two successive days for abdominal pain and on the second visit has an easily diagnosed appendiceal rupture, the chart that describes vigorous and concerted efforts to demonstrate peritoneal inflammation on the first visit indicates that, in all likelihood, nobody would have detected the appendicitis at that time. This is good practice of medicine for the patient and important protection for the physician.

Acute Appendicitis

Assessment

When trying to assess a difficult 5-year-old for appendicitis, the prime focus of the history taking and examination process must be on the attempt to demonstrate the presence of peritoneal inflammation in the right lower abdominal quadrant.

One soon recognizes that the act of approaching for the purpose of examining may be the single maneuver which, more than any other, upsets an already frightened child. However, the physical approach must be done at some stage; one way is to approach first and let the response settle down before having to lay hands on the child. If the physician places himself or herself close to the child, perhaps sitting casually on the edge of the stretcher right at the start, and takes the history from parents from that position, the child will soon believe that he or she is not yet being examined and may save any opposition until the examination begins. This permits the physician to examine surreptitiously while taking history, and when the time comes for palpation, the intimidation of the physical approach to the patient for examination has come and gone.

While eliciting history, and at the same time seeming to ignore the child, the examiner can watch the child out of the corner of his or her eye while "inadvertently" jiggling the stretcher. The child who at that instant clutches the right lower abdomen and cries out is demonstrating peritoneal irritation. Alternatively one can lay one's hand casually across the child's thigh and give it a familiar shake, in this way jiggling both thigh and pelvis. If the child indicates unexpected pain in the right lower abdomen, peritoneal irritation is present. When the more formal abdominal examination ends up as a total loss, as it sometimes does, information obtained through these initial "undercover" methods while taking history may prove to be the only useful information to be obtained on which decisions regarding the presence of peritoneal inflammation can be based.

Systemic symptoms are important in differentiating between appendicitis and generalized viral infections, many of which also have abdominal manifestations. Appendicitis remains well localized until perforation is imminent, and the presence of headache, fever, muscle aches and pains, chilly sensations, or dizziness at or near the onset of the illness favors a generalized infection.

Certain specific symptoms of acute appendicitis are of greater significance in children than in adults. Although an adult may not vomit but be merely anorectic for a day or so, the child under age 7 or 8 will almost certainly have vomited at least once. This symptom is so close to being absolute that the absence of vomiting in a 6-year-old (or younger) speaks strongly against appendicitis. Constipation is often taught as part of the history to be expected in appendicitis. However, the course of the disease in children is rarely long enough for there to be time for constipation to be recognized.

In the history-taking process, the focus is on seeking out indications of peritoneal inflammation. Questions need to be selected that satisfy this focus, but on the other hand, one should not lead. When asking about pain aggravated by movement, one should not just ask if the pain seemed to be worse when the child moved. One needs to discover if there seemed to be a stab of pain with every jiggle or jostle or, conversely, if the pain gradually got worse as the child was brought to the hospital.

Although abdominal examination is the crux of the evaluation of the child with abdominal pain, it is important also to assess the degree of systemic effects of the illness. Prior to perforation, the older child with acute appendicitis is unlikely to have much fever or tachycardia; nor is the child likely to be flushed or excessively pale. The younger child may have somewhat greater systemic manifestations, although these become much more marked when peritonitis develops.

The characteristics of respirations displayed by the child are often of diagnostic value. The child who has pain of either peritoneal or pleural origin is likely to grunt at the start of each expiration as he or she attempts to splint the diaphragm. A typical example of this is the 3-year-old who is brought to the hospital because of two or three days of abdominal pain and vomiting, who is whimpering but not vigorously crying because that hurts too much, who grunts with every breath, and who has a visibly distended abdomen. This child probably has general peritonitis from a ruptured appendix.

During the abdominal examination of a particularly anxious child, it is essential to use all one's wiles to distract the child's attention away from the examining hand. Capturing a frightened child's total attention can usually be accomplished with patience, and when it has been captured as much information as possible must be obtained before it is lost. For this reason, painful maneuvers must be left until the end.

When the child's attention is focused on the examiner's face, gentle abdominal palpation may demonstrate increased muscle tone. Exceedingly light pressure is required, though, so that the muscular resistance felt is truly reflex and not voluntary response to pain. Hyperesthesia is not of much value except in the older and completely cooperative individual.

At some stage the site of maximum tenderness must be located, and it is at this point that a degree of discomfort will inevitably be inflicted. If the patient's attention can be directed to the examiner's face and not the hand, the site of maximum tenderness can usually be found. While the conversation continues, gradually deepening pressure is exerted in the left lower, then the left upper, then the right upper, and lastly the right lower quadrants. If the examiner can be confident that he or she had the child's full attention, a sudden response indicating pain is very significant.

Although some argue that rectal examination is almost useless in children, nothing is further from the truth. Rectal examination reveals crucial information in enough cases that it is essential in all. Only when the need for a surgical consultation becomes obvious before the rectal examination is done may it be deferred until carried out by the surgeon. No patient seen for abdominal pain may be sent home as "not having appendicitis" without a rectal examination. As the least pleasant part of the examination, the rectal examination should be done last.

The child receiving a rectal examination should be on the back with the knees drawn up and spread apart, covered with a sheet. The child should not be lying on the side facing the wall. Nothing could be more frightening to an already anxious child than having to face the blank wall while someone he or she cannot see "attacks" from the rear. Face-to-face contact allows for explanations and reassurances. It also facilitates a "bimanual" form of examination because the examiner's left hand can feel the abdomen anteriorly, while the right index finger is in the rectum. There is probably no physical finding as useful in ruling out inflammation in the iliac fossae as the ability of the finger in the rectum to feel the outer hand as it moves (or vice versa) without severe discomfort.

When, after completion of the examination, the examiner still remains in doubt about the presence of peritoneal inflammation, several other steps may be taken to assist in ruling it out. The older child may be asked to stand and then to rise up several times onto the toes, each time pounding the heels back onto the floor. This should jolt the lower abdomen sufficiently to elicit pain from an inflamed appendix. The younger child may be asked to demonstrate what a good runner he or she is. Running to a parent down the hall is something most young children are usually happy to do unless doing so hurts.

Although some basic laboratory tests have become almost routine, they rarely do more than support the clinical impression. A polymorphonuclear leukocytosis is customary with acute suppurative appendicitis. However, a white cell count of 30,000 may be more suggestive of osteomyelitis or bacterial pneumonia than appendicitis. A low white cell count may imply exhaustion of defense mechanisms and the need for aggressive supportive therapy. Alternatively, it may suggest that the inflammation is viral in origin. Eradication of eosinophiles from the peripheral smear is almost as consistent an indicator of acute inflammatory disease as is neutrophilic leukocytosis.

Urinalysis may show white cells if there is a bacterial urinary infection. On the other hand, white cells may be present because an inflamed appendix lies close to the ureter. Ruling out glycosuria is an important preanesthetic step.

Routine abdominal radiography is not recommended in the assessment of a child with acute abdominal pain suspected to have acute appendicitis. In doubtful cases, the demonstration of a calcified fecalith has been claimed to be indication for operation. However, peritoneal irritation on examination remains the chief criterion.

If diagnosis is still in doubt, careful correlation of duration of the history, severity of symptoms, and magnitude of change in temperature and white cell count may weigh heavily for or against appendicitis. The child who has had pain for 4 days, has minimal abdominal findings, and has a normal temperature and white cell count almost certainly has something other than acute appendicitis. Similarly, the child with only a 6-hour history of abdominal pain, who is flushed and has a high temperature and white count, is more likely to have a systemic infection of some sort, in spite of the presence of some abdominal tenderness.

Even when all these diagnostic efforts are expended, doubt can still remain. In such cases, admission and repeated examinations over the next few hours may clarify the picture. Appendicitis is a progressive process, and one can expect it to show increasing manifestations as time passes. However, the observation period for a child should be strictly limited. If the situation cannot be resolved within 10 or 12 hours, many would proceed to laparotomy as an alternative safer than observing any longer and risking perforation with its complications.

Treatment

For all cases a surgical opinion should be requested. The proper treatment for early or unruptured appendicitis is emergency appendectomy. Although complicated cases such as those demonstrating generalized peritonitis will need skillful medical, anesthetic, and surgical care, the principle of treatment is still removal of the ruptured organ. The peritoneal space tolerates one brief contamination surprisingly well. It does not tolerate well continuing fecal soilage.

When the peritoneal space is first opened, several liters of fluid are usually noted to gush from the abdominal cavity of any child with appendiceal perforation and general peritonitis. This volume of liquid has been lost and emphasizes the need for fluid resuscitation prior to operation. Fluid resuscitation should be started in the emergency department with Ringer's lactate or physiologic saline while the surgeon is awaited.

Intussusception

Assessment

The classic textbook history of intussusception is that of a 5- to 10-month-old infant who has had a few hours of intermittent screaming spells, pulling up of the legs with each pain, perhaps vomiting, and possibly the passage of a "currant jelly stool."

The pain itself is due to small bowel obstruction and is an intestinal colic. In 70 to 80 percent of instances, the intermittent pain is the chief presenting complaint, and in another 5 to 10 percent, although not the presenting complaint, there is intermittent pain elicited on questioning. In about 10 to 15 percent, particularly in the first 2 to 4 months of life, pain is not a major feature of the disease, although the infant will generally be quite irritable.

Vomiting occurs in about 25 to 30 percent, especially if there has been a recent feeding. This symptom is of particular importance in infants in the first few months of life. Rectal bleeding is not as common now as it was decades ago when medical care was less apt to be sought promptly. The classically described currant jelly stool is an admixture of mucus, blood, and stool and has a variety of consistencies and hues depending on the relative proportions of the constituents.

Intussusception in the 2- or 3-month-old infant usually has a different course from that of the 7-month-old infant. Abdominal pain is much less characteristic; the tiny baby with an intussusception will usually have vomiting and irritability as the prime symptoms.

On examination the infant will often manifest an unusual grayish type of pallor, which is frequently described by more senior clinicians, although it is less often recognized now. Unless the condition has been present for more than a day or so, the baby can be expected to be vigorous and active. The picture of shock is unusual, unless peritonitis, an unexpected complication of intussusception, has developed or the amount of rectal bleeding has been much greater than is customary.

Abdominal palpation will, in 60 to 70 percent of instances, reveal a nontender, tubular mass, oriented transversely and located in the mid or right upper abdomen. The mass will be situated deeply against the posterior abdominal wall because the mesentery will have been pulled into the intussuscipiens as the intussusceptum moves ahead. Rectal examination may reveal blood in the rectum or on the examining finger, or, rarely, the leading end of the mass may be low enough to be palpable within the lumen of the rectum. In the very rare instance, the intussusceptum may even prolapse out through the anus.

Atypical presentations are common. In the very young infant, usually under 4 months of age, pain is less of a feature and is replaced by vomiting and rectal bleeding as the chief presenting symptoms. Bloody diarrhea can be very misleading when it is the presenting symptom for an intussusception. Gastroenteritis is the most common admitting diagnosis to be subsequently changed to intussusception.

Intussusception is seen more often in the child over 3 years of age than was previously thought. In the older child, the history is generally less acute than is seen in the infant, with several days of colic frequently preceding any other symptoms.

Although the majority of intussusceptions are idiopathic, 10 to 15 percent have as a predisposing cause an organic lesion in the small bowel, the most common of these being a Meckel's diverticulum. It has been generally observed that hydrostatic reduction of the intussusception is very unlikely to succeed when there is an underlying organic cause. Thus, there is little reason to fear that an intussusception caused by a Meckel's diverticulum might be reduced hydrostatically and the underlying lesion missed.

Confirmation of the diagnosis requires radiographic demonstration of the lesion by means of a contrast enema. Although traditionally the barium enema was widely used, many centers currently use air as the contrast medium.

In many centers, plain films of the abdomen are routine for all patients in whom bowel obstruction is considered to be a possibility. However, virtually the only cause of acute bowel obstruction in infancy is intussusception and, although plain films can be suggestive, intussusception is not confirmed by them. Hence, unless the radiologist demands a plain film to rule out free intraperitoneal air, something that can be obtained at the start of the contrast enema procedure, there is no reason to think plain films should play any part in the initial work-up of a baby thought to have an intussusception. It is more logical to avoid the unnecessary radiation and the delay plain films introduce and to proceed directly to the contrast study.

Treatment

The definitive treatment of intussusception in at least 70 percent of instances is hydrostatic reduction. Hence, the confirmatory diagnostic measure becomes the definitive therapy in a majority of cases. Although most babies are seen early enough now that they are in excellent condition when they go to the radiology department for a contrast enema, intussusception is a form of small bowel obstruction and fluid loss eventually becomes part of the clinical picture. Therefore, the need for fluid resuscitation before anything else is done should be kept in mind, particularly in the young baby under 5 months of age.

The compromised bowel in an intussusception is within the colon and does not tend to produce either the peritoneal signs or the systemic toxicity that would be expected with ischemic bowel exposed in the coelom. Because peritoneal signs do not develop as bowel becomes compromised, there is no dependable clinical way of estimating the stage of the disease. Hence, the very information that is needed to avoid hydrostatically reducing dead bowel is not available. However, it has been shown both clinically and experimentally that, except in the very rare instance, hydrostatic reduction, using carefully controlled pressures, will not reduce necrotic bowel because of the fibrinous adhesions which gradually form about the neck of the intussusception as ischemic changes progress.

When attempted hydrostatic reduction fails, the child is taken directly to the operating theater for laparotomy and manual reduction of the intussusception. Incidental appendectomy is usually carried out, although there is little thought nowadays that the appendix plays any part in the etiology of the telescoping.

If dead bowel is encountered at operation, or when the telescoping cannot be manually reduced without tearing the bowel wall, the whole segment is resected.

Other Causes of Acute Abdominal Pain

Obstructive Causes

Adhesive Bowel Obstruction

The child who has had previous abdominal surgery and who complains of acute abdominal pain and vomiting should be assumed to have an adhesive small bowel obstruction and must be evaluated at once with this condition in mind. When a loop of bowel becomes caught around a postoperative adhesion and undergoes a volvulus, venous infarction of that loop is rapid and serious. Apart from trauma, a closed loop bowel obstruction around an adhesion is almost the only abdominal condition in childhood that can result in critical illness and even death in a surprisingly few hours. Particularly in the younger child, but to a comparable degree in all children, the progression of toxicity can be fulminant and lead to gram-positive sepsis and shock within a few hours.

The symptoms of adhesive small bowel obstruction are intermittent intestinal cramps and vomiting, which becomes bilious early on and perhaps even feculent in time. Failure to pass stool or gas will be noted eventually, although not until the bowel below the obstruction has emptied. The characteristic physical findings are a distended and tympanitic abdomen, a succussion splash, and, most diagnostic of all, a high-pitched peristaltic "tinkle" synchronous with each pain. Associated symptoms and signs of peritoneal irritation imply the presence of bowel with a compromised blood supply.

Radiographs usually reveal multiple gas-filled loops of small bowel arranged transversely (ladder pattern) and a dearth of stool or gas in the colon. Urgent surgical consultation is warranted because of the potential for rapid deterioration. Intravenous resuscitation should be begun immediately because fluid losses into the abdominal cavity can be in alarming volumes.

Midgut Volvulus with Underlying Incomplete Midgut Rotation

The neonate or young infant with incomplete midgut rotation, commonly called malrotation, is usually in enough trouble in the first few weeks of life from duodenal obstruction that the diagnosis is made and the rotational anomaly is corrected surgically. However, every so often the duodenal obstruction is not a major factor early on and the baby survives, seemingly healthy, into childhood with the midgut still suspended on a narrow pedicle that is prone to twist.

Episodes of midgut volvulus in childhood usually occur as attacks of recurrent abdominal pain, which may go undiagnosed for many months until a more severe attack leads to investigation, diagnosis, and appropriate treatment. Ideally the underlying anomaly is diagnosed and treated on the basis of mild recurrent episodes. Unfortunately, this is not always the case, and rare instances do occur in which the first presentation is that of severe bowel obstruction and shock caused by midgut infarction. Even in these instances, one is likely to elicit a history of milder episodes for which medical attention was not sought.

The clinical picture of midgut volvulus is that of severe intestinal obstruction with distention and bilious vomiting. Rapid deterioration in general condition and increasing indication of peritoneal irritation parallel the process of intestinal necrosis. This is a highly lethal condition, and the only effective therapy is early surgical exploration and correction of the volvulus in the hope that there will be enough small bowel remaining viable to subserve nutritional requirements. When there is doubt regarding the amount of bowel remaining that will be functional, some surgeons leave all intestine in place after reducing the volvulus with the plan to re-explore in 48 hours, at which time clearer demarcation of the infarcted bowel may be evident. This may permit more bowel to be preserved than would have been the case had resection been carried out primarily.

In spite of the dramatic nature of the volvulus and its high mortality rate, most patients with underlying incomplete midgut rotation will be seen on a number of occasions because of recurrent milder attacks of pain. Consequently, this condition is also discussed in some detail under chronic or recurrent abdominal pain (Chapter 19).

Meckel's Band

When the embryonic vitelline fistula fails to resorb completely, it may leave a variety of forms of remnants. Although a Meckel's diverticulum alone is the most common vitelline remnant, a persisting fibrous band between the tip of the diverticulum and the umbilicus (a Meckel's band) is also seen from time to time and may act in similar fashion to a postoperative adhesion around which a loop of bowel can twist. An infant who presents with an acute small bowel obstruction probably has an intussusception. However, when the contrast enema has ruled out an ileocolic intussusception in such an infant, the intestinal obstruction is very likely to be caused by a Meckel's band.

Incarcerated Inguinal Hernia

In the third world countries, incarcerated or strangulated inguinal hernias are still important causes of acute intestinal obstruction. In contrast, in areas where pediatric care is of good quality, inguinal hernias, particularly in infancy, are routinely repaired soon after diagnosis, and the chief complications, namely incarceration and strangulation, are uncommon. Furthermore, hernias that have become incarcerated are customarily seen and treated well before the stage of intestinal obstruction ensues.

Miscellaneous Causes of Acute Intestinal Obstruction

Internal hernias through congenital mesenteric defects are rare and diagnosed at operation carried out for small bowel obstruction. With travel becoming so prevalent throughout the world and with so many families of different racial origins emigrating to larger cities in the Western world, diseases endemic in tropical areas are being seen more often. Roundworm infestations, so common in Africa and in the Mediterranean area, are not often of surgical importance. However, emergency operation can be required to treat either intestinal obstruction caused by an intraluminal bolus of intertwined roundworms or, much less commonly, peritonitis resulting from roundworm perforation.

In the fibrocystic child, a degree of obstruction is rarely seen to arise from impaction of abnormally inspissated intestinal contents in the ileocecal area (''meconium ileus equivalent''). This can usually be handled by colonic administration of enemas containing acetylcysteine.

Foreign body ingestion can on occasion result in obstruction. Some children have the habit of eating unshelled sunflower seeds. Although the risk of problems arising from the ingestion of small amounts is negligible, when taken in large amounts a bolus of the shells can sometimes form in the rectum, where it can be felt as a hard ball with multiple sharp protuberances on the surface. If this is large enough, it will not only obstruct, but also cannot be passed by the child. The only kind way to handle this situation is disimpaction under general anesthesia.

Although constipation does not cause the symptoms of acute intestinal obstruction, a form of it can cause acute abdominal pain that may simulate an abdominal surgical emergency. This is discussed under nonsurgical causes of abdominal pain. Severe functional constipation of long duration may cause abdominal distention and overflow leakage or encopresis. However, this is clearly a chronic situation. In addition, pain is not an important feature of this state, nor is it of Hirschsprung's disease, the chief condition from which severe functional constipation must be differentiated.

Inflammatory Causes

Ovarian Lesions

Postpubertal girls may display the same abdominal episodes of pain as their elders, whether due to bleeding from a graafian follicle following ovulation (mittelschmerz) or from a persisting corpus luteum during or immediately after menses. The same diagnostic quandary can be encountered in the younger mature female as in the older, and in some doubtful cases laparoscopy is used to assist in the differentiation.

On the other hand, appendicitis is a common disease in the teenage and young adult years, and in view of the serious danger of sterility as a result of lower abdominal peritonitis in the female, surgeons justifiably are more aggressive in exploring such abdomens when appendicitis cannot be excluded with complete confidence.

Torsion of an ovarian cyst or solid tumor in the child is as unusual as the overall incidence of ovarian tumors in childhood would suggest. However, acute pain and marked indication of peritoneal irritation in a lower quadrant and adnexal region must include an ovarian catastrophe as a strong possibility. Those occurring on the right are usually discovered at exploration for appendicitis. Those on the left have a chance at a more accurate diagnosis with the help of ultrasonography or, if necessary, computed tomographic scan.

Primary Peritonitis

Primary peritonitis arises without any gastrointestinal or other perforation to provide the contamination and, therefore, is thought to develop because of organisms that have reached the abdominal cavity via blood or lymphatic channels. Although relatively rare in previously well children, it is quite common in the nephrotic child.

The previously completely well child developing primary peritonitis is most likely to be a 3- to 8-year-old girl with one or two days' history of steady lower abdominal pain, subsequently becoming aggravated by movement, and vomiting.

On examination there will be the findings of lower abdominal peritonitis, although all the maneuvers described under acute appendicitis to assist in the abdominal examination may be required to demonstrate it. Although one cannot with certainty differentiate primary peritonitis from perforated appendicitis, the observation may be made that the child with primary peritonitis is less toxic, has not vomited as often, and may not have as marked abdominal signs. Nevertheless, in the child who has been previously completely healthy and who has not had an appendectomy in the past, findings that point to lower abdominal peritonitis must be assumed to be due to appendiceal rupture until laparotomy has demonstrated otherwise.

Generally, the diagnosis of primary peritonitis is made at operation for presumed acute appendicitis. There will be a turbid peritoneal exudate, most marked in the lower abdomen and the pouch of Douglas, with mild serositis of those parts of the bowel which have been in contact with the exudate. This includes the appendix, although the appendix will not be inflamed to any greater degree than the rest of the intestine. The absence of any localized bowel pathology, perforation or otherwise, establishes this as a primary form of peritonitis.

Culture of the exudate reveals a pure bacterial growth in most cases, usually of an *Escherichia coli* strain, or alternatively pneumococcus or *Streptococcus*. Other organisms reported are exceedingly rare. Appropriate antibiotic therapy results in rapid recovery.

Primary peritonitis is a common complication of the nephrotic syndrome, whether in remission or relapse. Hence, when a child being seen for abdominal pain, known to be nephrotic, is found to have generalized lower abdominal peritonitis, it is justified to make the diagnosis of primary peritonitis. However, this diagnosis is no more than presumptive until prompt response to intravenous antibiotic therapy is noted over the next 8 to 12 hours. Primary peritonitis associated with nephrosis is usually due to a pneumococcus, or less often *Streptococcus*. Hence, the antibiotic selected is customarily penicillin. If a marked response is not promptly noted, consideration must be given to immediate exploration with the diagnosis of perforated appendicitis.

Nephrotic or other renal patients being managed on continuous peritoneal dialysis are even more prone to bacterial peritonitis. In this situation, irrigation of the peritoneal space through the dialysis catheter, in addition to intravenous antibiotic therapy, leads to prompt resolution of the infection.

Meckel's Diverticulitis

Because of the appendix-like form of a Meckel's diverticulum, there is a theoretic possibility of obstruction at its base and subsequent inflammation distal to the obstruction, akin to the appendicitis process. This is often quoted as a possible cause of acute abdominal pain comparable to that of appendicitis but more likely to be situated in the left lower abdominal quadrant.

Inflammation is a most unusual way for a Meckel's diverticulum to occur. Hemorrhage and intestinal obstruction account for almost all the clinical cases in which pathology of a Meckel's diverticulum has caused illness. However, rare as it is, diverticulitis is a theoretic possibility and is reported from time to time. Therefore, the surgeon will need to be aware of it should the condition be encountered when exploring because of progressive signs of peritoneal inflammation.

Crohn's Disease

Granulomatous enteritis is well known for its ability to cause acute episodes of lower abdominal pain and tenderness that can simulate acute appendicitis. In addition, there may or may not be a palpable mass. In most cases, there will be a past history of cramps or other indication of episodes of incomplete obstruction. Nevertheless, when a child known to have Crohn's disease has for the first time an episode of right lower quadrant pain, it can be impossible to make the differentiation without direct inspection of the appendix, small bowel, or both at operation.

Inguinoscrotal Lesions

One important result of insisting on a rectal examination carried out in the supine position for abdominal pain is that it presents the external genitalia for inspection. This reminder is important. Rarely a young child will complain of abdominal pain but in reality have an incarcerated inguinal hernia, torsion of a testis, or torsion of an appendix testis. When seeking the cause of acute abdominal pain, the physician must always remember to examine the inguinoscrotal area.

Miscellaneous Medical Conditions Causing Acute Abdominal Pain

Constipation

A well-recognized syndrome of fecal accumulation in the sigmoid colon appears with intermittent mid and left lower quadrant pain, left lower quadrant tenderness, occasionally mild indication of peritoneal irritation, and, from time to time, a palpable mass. The patient is usually from 5 to 15 years of age and may or may not have a history of constipation. This condition can begin with such severe pains and display such marked tenderness and peritoneal irritation which is so definite that the diagnosis of appendicitis would be automatic were it to develop on the right side.

When pain and tenderness are localized to the left lower quadrant, one is well advised to assess the effect of a small enema before trying anything else. In most instances, the enema will produce clear therapeutic benefit. The pain and tenderness will disappear, and abdominal examination will usually then be normal. This therapeutic "trial" will, in most instances, render unnecessary any radiographs, other investigations, or expensive consultations. An enema not only establishes the diagnosis, but also treats the condition.

If an enema does not improve the clinical picture, no harm will have been done by it, and one can then give any needed consideration to other causes of left lower quadrant pain and tenderness, such as atypical appendicitis, ovarian pathology, primary peritonitis, and viral illness.

Viral Flu-Like Illnesses with Abdominal Components

Generalized viral infections frequently cause abdominal pain. Although the pain is often crampy, it may have the characteristics of appendicitis with a steady component associated with tenderness and some peritoneal irritation. When such a child is operated on for presumed acute appendicitis, one usually finds the terminal small bowel and appendix to be slightly inflamed and the mesentery to be edematous. In the peritoneal space, there may be a small amount of clear watery fluid, which may grow the virus.

Because the lymph nodes in the mesentery may be somewhat enlarged and inflamed in this condition, it is often labeled mesenteric adenitis. However, it is preferable to save the term mesenteric adenitis for those cases of marked enlargement of the iliocecal mesenteric nodes that is occasionally discovered at operation carried out for presumed appendicitis and that is usually due to *Yersinia enterocolitica*.

Although differentiating a viral flu from acute appendicitis may be very difficult, one can usually make the differentiation by considering that the viral infection is basically a systemic infection that can then involve the lower abdomen, whereas appendicitis is primarily a local process in the right lower abdomen that can later produce some systemic manifestations. Illness that has chills, headache, fever and muscle pains first and then has abdominal pain is probably a systemic infection with subsequent abdominal inflammation. When the initial symptom is midabdominal cramps, followed by right lower quadrant pain and tenderness, and then still later fever and tachycardia of a generalized process, one thinks more of appendicitis, which begins in the organ itself and produces systemic signs later.

The child with influenza is usually flushed and perhaps dizzy when asked to stand up. The child may be perspiring and probably has a mild tachycardia. Such a child usually looks ill. The child with as yet unruptured appendicitis generally looks well and rarely has much in the way of systemic manifestations.

The white cell count in a viral infection is variable, although early on granulocytic leukocytosis is common. When seen in the hospital for abdominal pain, leukopenia is often noted. Clearly one cannot place too much emphasis on the white cell count: it is supportive evidence only, not diagnostic.

Treatment for a child with abdominal pain who is presumed to have a viral infection as the underlying illness is based on the fact that the diagnosis remains presumptive until the course of the illness confirms it. Consequently, the focus of treatment is continued close follow-up in case atypical appendicitis becomes evident.

Gastroenteritis

Cramps and diarrhea in combination will, in most instances, be sufficient to establish the diagnosis of gastroenteritis, usually viral, occasionally bacterial. However, before the diarrhea begins, cramps alone introduce concerns regarding the possibility of intussusception, early appendicitis, or other less dramatic conditions. However, with the onset of acute nonbloody diarrhea, intussusception and appendicitis become highly unlikely or can be ruled out, although an acutely inflamed appendix adjacent to the sigmoid colon or rectum can result in a mucoid discharge that might be interpreted as diarrhea.

Bloody diarrhea, particularly in infancy, must bring intussusception to mind, and any infant being treated for gastroenteritis who has blood in diarrheal stools must be watched very closely. Failure to respond quickly to treatment requires that intussusception again be ruled out. When infants who are shown ultimately to have intussusception have been admitted with an incorrect diagnosis, that diagnosis has usually been gastroenteritis.

"Green-Apple Tummy"

Abdominal pain after dietary indiscretion can usually be identified for what it is on the basis of dietary history and the lack of physical findings. When there are suspicious abdominal findings, a few hours of observation will usually settle the issue in view of the self-limiting nature of the illness.

Urinary Tract Infections

Urinary infections from time to time do cause enough abdominal pain that intraperitoneal disease must be excluded. Urinalysis will generally establish the diagnosis, particularly if there are pus cell casts indicating acute pyelonephritis. On the other hand, a few white cells in the urine do not exclude appendicitis because this finding can be produced by an acutely inflamed appendix adjacent to the ureter or bladder.

In addition, even when there is pyuria to a degree clearly indicative of a urinary infection, definite signs of peritoneal inflammation over the appendiceal area must be given serious consideration even to the extent of exploration. Appendicitis and urinary infections are both fairly common diseases, and the presence of one does not exclude the other.

Pneumonia

Lung infections occasionally result in the picture of abdominal pain, presumably as a result of phrenic involvement. Grunting is an important clue to peritoneal pain, particularly in infants. Grunting can also be due to pleural pain, when it is really an attempt to minimize pain by splinting the diaphragm. The history of a cough in the previous few days, rapid breathing, and visible nasal flaring should alert the physician to the possibility of pneumonia. A chest radiograph will confirm or exclude the diagnosis, although a lateral projection is needed to discover an area of retrocardiac consolidation. Indeed, in the young child a chest film is frequently much more useful in the investigation of acute abdominal pain than is abdominal radiography.

Diabetes Mellitus

Diabetic children who have periodic episodes of ketoacidosis may complain of abdominal pain during the course of an episode. Indeed, on occasion there may be some features of an acute surgical abdomen. However, the differentiation is usually not difficult to make because there is rapid improvement with correction of the ketoacidotic state.

When the abdominal pain of ketoacidosis occurs in a child not previously known to be diabetic, there can be diagnostic confusion until the glucosuria and hyperglycemia are recognized. This is only one of the reasons for the need to test urine for glucose prior to emergency anesthesia.

Rheumatic Fever

Historically rheumatic fever is rarely said to cause abdominal pain before the onset of any of the other characteristics that identify the true nature of the illness. Experience with one such case in which abdominal pain preceded a swollen ankle by several hours hardly qualifies the author as an expert on the condition. However, it is clear that abdominal pain can be present with the onset of rheumatic fever, and where rheumatic fever occurs with a significant frequency, this needs to be kept in mind.

CHAPTER

19

Recurrent Abdominal Pain

General Considerations

Recurrent abdominal pain is a common complaint. Many children miss school repeatedly; see various physicians including family practitioners, pediatricians, psychiatrists, and surgeons; undergo endless investigations and even operations all in an effort to find the cause of recurrent attacks of abdominal pain. In a majority of such children no organic cause is ever found, and the diagnoses assigned vary from "functional abdominal pain" or "school phobia" to frank "malingering."

The emergency department is not the proper environment in which to evaluate and investigate a child who has been intermittently missing school or other activities because of recurrent abdominal pain. Such a child needs a detailed, careful, comprehensive assessment away from the excitement and activity of the emergency department. However, the child with recurrent pain is sometimes encountered in the department, possibly because the present attack "seemed much worse," the child had not had an attack for a month or so and "something must have happened to bring another one on," or "the doctor said he couldn't tell what was going on unless he saw him in an attack."

The obligation of emergency department staff when seeing this type of patient is to ensure that the present attack is similar to all other attacks and that there is nothing different about it to indicate an acute surgical emergency and to ensure that the child is under the care of a physician who is proceeding with or has carried out appropriate work-up to find the cause. Emergency department staff should resist the temptation to take a 45-minute history, do a complete physical examination, and embark on radiographic studies when there is no indication that emergency care is needed. The assessment of this type of complaint must be by someone who not only can do it thoroughly, but also can ensure continuity of care.

However, to have the confidence to be able to say, "there is no emergency at the present time, so you can go back to your own physician," the emergency physician must be aware of some of the facts about this clinical problem.

Although most recurrent abdominal pain in children is not due to organic disease, several serious surgical conditions can cause recurrent pain and may be readily missed for a disturbingly long time unless they are kept in mind. There is always danger of such a child acquiring a psychiatric or behavioral label early on; when a diagnosis, however ill-founded, has been assigned, one does not tend to remain open-minded about other possibilities.

It is interesting that recurrent abdominal pain is more likely to be due to important organic disease when it occurs in the young child than when it occurs in the teenager.

Specific Causes of Recurrent Pains

The organic lesions that can cause recurrent abdominal pains are many and varied. However, those few which are of a sufficiently emergent nature to require prompt treatment in the emergency department are restricted to conditions involving the intestine, the urinary tract, and, in the adolescent girl, the ovary.

Intestinal Lesions

The sort of intestinal conditions to be considered are those which can cause intermittent bowel obstruction, particularly involving small bowel. The most important one, and the one most urgently in need of being ruled out in this situation, is recurrent midgut volvulus in the child with an underlying embryonic incomplete midgut rotation (malrotation). If the child has undergone previous thorough work-up, this will presumably have been ruled out by radiographic investigation. However, if it has not and there are signs of peritoneal irritation to imply compromise of intestinal blood supply, malrotation is a strong possibility. Conversely, even if there are no abdominal findings at the moment, if malrotation has not been ruled out by contrast studies, one should make sure that such studies are planned for the near future. This is one radiologic study which the emergency physician might feel justified in ordering for a patient with recurrent abdominal pain. Midgut volvulus is almost the only condition from which the child might conceivably become critically ill within a few hours. Missing this diagnosis can lead to a fatality.

Intermittent incomplete small bowel obstruction from a congenital Meckel's band is also a possibility, but one cannot expect to diagnose it by radiographic means, although a pertechnetate nuclear study may reveal the presence of a Meckel's diverticulum (Meckel's scan). This may be found only when the child's abdomen is being explored for intestinal obstruction. The infant with a small bowel obstruction who is thought to have an intussusception but has a normal emergency contrast enema quite likely has a Meckel's band as the cause of obstruction.

Other organic causes of incomplete small bowel obstruction, such as tumors of the bowel, may be demonstrable on computed tomographic scan but for the most part will be discovered only at operation for obstruction.

Urinary Lesions

Urinary tract infections, or congenital obstructive lesions, can cause abdominal pains of an intermittent nature. These do not appear generally as emergencies but should be included in the possibilities to be looked for.

Ovarian Lesions

When the young girl is operated on for torsion of an ovarian tumor, one may elicit the history that there have been previous attacks of pain that were milder but otherwise similar to the pain of the twisted tumor. Consequently, when attacks of pain are localized to one side, an organic lesion should be carefully looked for, with special thought to the possibility of recurrent torsion of an ovarian tumor.

Other Organic Causes

Other organic causes of recurrent pain range from the commonplace, such as chronic constipation, to the rare, such as porphyria. The pediatric neurologist adds abdominal migraine and abdominal epilepsy to the list of causes of recurrent abdominal pain, although both are distinctly rare and require sophisticated neurologic consultation and investigation to establish. At any rate, when the emergency physician can be confident that there is no acute surgical emergency present, little further effort to identify the culprit is warranted in the emergency context.

20

Gastrointestinal Bleeding

General Considerations

Some general features of bleeding from the gastrointestinal tract need review before specific bleeding lesions are discussed.

The possibility of a bleeding diathesis must always be considered when either gastric or rectal bleeding is encountered. For this reason, vitamin K deficiency, hemophilia in one form or another, and thrombocytopenia all need to be remembered when history is being taken, and the appropriate blood studies need to be done unless there is clear evidence for a specific organic lesion which is bleeding.

Red or black stools usually lead to the belief that the child is "bleeding." However, fresh blood and old changed blood are not the only substances that turn feces red and black, respectively. Beets and certain antibiotics or other drugs are examples of the several categories of materials taken by mouth that can stain stools red. Iron and licorice, among other substances, are known to produce black stools. When there is any doubt that the discoloration is due to blood, one of the simple chemical tests for blood should be used as verification.

In the case of the neonate, maternal blood ingested during the delivery can show up many hours postpartum when the infant either vomits or passes it through the rectum. In addition, the breast-fed baby may ingest maternal blood from cracked or tender nipples. Before a source of bleeding is sought, the presence of fetal hemoglobin should be confirmed by the use of one of the simple tests available (e.g., the Apt test). In the neonate or the young breast-fed baby, the absence of fetal hemoglobin indicates the blood to be of maternal origin.

Upper gastrointestinal hemorrhage, arbitrarily defined as coming from the esophagus, stomach, or duodenum, is generally characterized by hematemesis. Lower gastrointestinal hemorrhage, from jejunum or more distal bowel, rarely if ever refluxes far enough to produce vomiting of blood. When in doubt, the examination of gastric aspirate obtained through a nasogastric tube is instrumental in differentiating an upper gastrointestinal hemorrhage from a lower gastrointestinal hemorrhage. Only rarely will a source of bleeding in the duodenum fail to result in reflux of blood into the stomach.

Associated symptoms may reveal the diagnosis, such as the cramps of an intussusception or the diarrhea of bacterial enteritis. In such cases, the rectal bleeding is not the chief complaint and may be only incidental. In other cases, the age of the patient provides an important clue to the probable diagnosis.

Sometimes the bleeding itself is of such a magnitude that resuscitative measures are necessary before any thought can be given to looking for a cause. When surgical intervention is required to stop bleeding before there is time for any sophisticated investigation, an experienced, educated guess as to the cause of the bleeding can be critical.

There is a major philosophical difference between children and adults in the handling of undiagnosed rectal bleeding. In children several basic investigative tests are appropriate after an episode of bleeding. However, unless the bleeding continues or occurs a number of times, operation is not often indicated; this results in a number of children having had one or two episodes of rectal hemorrhage without any definitive diagnosis ever being made. This is in sharp contrast to adults, in whom the strong possibility of carcinoma makes almost mandatory the obtaining of an etiologic diagnosis after as little as one episode, even if it requires exploratory surgery to do so.

In this chapter, emphasis is given to two uniquely pediatric causes of painless and otherwise asymptomatic bleeding from the rectum. These are characteristic examples of, respectively, massive bleeding in infancy and painless spotting in the older child. Other pediatric causes of gastrointestinal hemorrhage are also covered but in less detail.

Bleeding Meckel's Diverticulum

The most common form of remnant persisting because of incomplete obliteration of the embryonic vitelline fistula, or omphalomesenteric duct, is a Meckel's diverticulum. This is situated along the antimesenteric border of the ileum at the site of the termination of the superior mesenteric artery (embryonic midpoint of the midgut) and frequently possesses gastric mucous membrane as at least part of its inner covering. The acid-pepsin secreted by this mucosa may cause peptic ulceration near the base of the diverticulum, where the mucous membrane is that of normal ileum, or in the ileum itself adjacent to the diverticulum. When the ulceration erodes into a blood vessel, the volume of hemorrhage can be comparable to the most actively bleeding peptic ulcer encountered in adult practice.

Active hemorrhage from a Meckel's diverticulum usually occurs in the first 2 years of life and produces the picture of a happy, unconcerned, but increasingly pale baby filling diaper after diaper with red blood. Examination rarely reveals anything diagnostic, although the degree of vasoconstriction may be striking and indicates active compensation to major blood loss.

While examining the baby, the physician should be alert to indications of abdominal pain, which might suggest intussusception, although in this lesion cramps usually take preeminence over hemorrhage except from time to time in the very young infant. Sites of bruising should be sought lest a bleeding diathesis be missed. Cutaneous hemangiomas should be noted as possible indicators of multiple vascular malformations, perhaps even involving bowel, although these are rare. Intestinal duplications that communicate with the bowel lumen and hence may bleed and massive hemorrhage from gastroduodenal ulcerations are also rare. Hence, the probability that the above picture is produced by a bleeding Meckel's diverticulum is very high.

A pertechnetate Meckel's nuclear scan is a useful investigative tool on an elective or semielective basis. However, when faced with an infant who is bleeding massively from the rectum and will require laparotomy in spite of a negative Meckel's scan, the delay introduced by proceeding with the test is not likely warranted. On the other hand, when an active hemorrhage stops spontaneously, removing the need for emergency surgery, an elective scan may be very worthwhile.

Because of the experience so important in the resuscitation of an infant in shock, the judgment needed when deciding to operate on an emergency basis, and the anesthetic expertise required during the procedure, referral before the baby is in serious physiologic difficulty is essential.

Juvenile Polyps

The term "juvenile polyps" is applied to colonic polyps seen in children, which are usually pedunculated, generally restricted to the colon, and for the most part asymptomatic except for rectal spotting of bright red blood. Juvenile polyps are the most common cause of spotting of blood from a rectal lesion in childhood. The blood appears on the stool or is expressed immediately after the stool, which is itself otherwise completely normal.

Examination rarely reveals anything abnormal. The lesion itself is generally either too soft or too high to be palpable in the rectum. No fissure is to be seen, and the stool is not unduly hard.

For practical purposes, rectal bleeding from polyps is restricted to children over the age of 2. Conversely, rectal bleeding in a child under the age of 2 is almost never due to polyps.

Polyps rarely bleed vigorously enough to require emergency treatment. Therefore, elective investigation is usually embarked on to confirm the diagnosis. Because endoscopy in the young child usually requires general anesthesia, radiographic studies are generally carried out first. This entails double contrast enema with postevacuation studies and requires a carefully prepared colon for satisfactory visualization, something often difficult to achieve in children.

Several or more polyps may be present in the one colon (multiple polyps), although only the ones in the sigmoid colon and lower are prone to bleed because of trauma from the harder and drier stool distally.

With very few exceptions, juvenile polyps display under the microscope an inner stroma of interlacing fibrous tissue strands around dilated glands. All this is enclosed within a thin basement membrane and a mucous membrane that consists of normal colonic mucosa showing attenuation and erosion, presumably where it has been subjected to superficial trauma. Erosions on the surface are the source of bleeding.

The basic difference between the histopathology of a juvenile polyp and that of the adult adenomatous polyp must be emphasized. The adult adenoma is a proliferative, epithelial neoplasm with precancerous potential. The juvenile polyp is not an epithelial lesion and has no premalignant tendency. The lack of any long-term concern regarding development of carcinoma removes not only the need for surgical treatment of juvenile polyps that are not producing symptoms, but also the need for continual re-examinations as the years pass.

Polyps that bleed are almost always within the range of the conventional sigmoidoscope. Polyps higher up rarely cause symptoms, and it is now recognized that they can be left where they are, although increasing facility with the colonoscope may affect this policy in the future. In some children, contrast enemas carried out because of rectal bleeding may demonstrate a number of polyps distributed throughout the colon. In such a case, almost certainly there is at least one polyp in the rectum or low sigmoid, within reach of the sigmoidoscope, which is the one that has been bleeding, and after this has been removed by electric snare technique through the endoscope, the others should cause no further symptoms.

As a result of this policy not to remove asymptomatic polyps, there are many juvenile polyps which remain in the colons of older children and teenagers and are never resected. In spite of this, surgeons rarely if ever see juvenile polyps in adults. When late follow-up contrast enemas are performed on older teenagers who had several polyps previously diagnosed but left in situ, it becomes apparent that polyps disappear spontaneously if permitted to do so, presumably by twisting and becoming detached. By adult life, all juvenile polyps have pretty well disappeared.

We know that the tendency for the polyps to be avulsed is also present in the younger child because from time to time the child with a good history for polyp, or with a previously diagnosed but as yet untreated polyp, will unexpectedly have a brisk intestinal hemorrhage and will then pass the polyp through the rectum. Alternatively, although the child may describe having passed a piece of tissue with the blood, sometimes there is no recognition of passing the polyp, even though the diagnosis seems pretty clear from history alone. Although one prefers not to subject a child to general anesthesia without a confirmed diagnosis, on occasion a child arrives bleeding briskly from what is presumed to be the stalk of an avulsed polyp. Fortunately such a hemorrhage usually stops spontaneously. When it does not, the surgeon can be in the position of having to perform sigmoidoscopy under general anesthesia for the purpose of cauterizing the bleeding stalk of an avulsed polyp, with a diagnosis based on history alone.

Trauma

Serious closed trauma to the abdomen does not generally cause significant intestinal hemorrhage because the bleeding that does occur is from solid organ rupture and therefore is into the peritoneal space. Uncommonly, traces of blood can be passed, presumably as incidental results of intestinal contusion, but are of little importance relative to the other injuries. However, whenever significant rectal bleeding is encountered following blunt abdominal trauma, consideration must be given to laceration of bowel, a lesion which should also be suggested by the rest of the examination.

Sometimes rectal bleeding will be the presenting complaint in a child who, on investigation, reveals that he or she, or someone else, has inserted a foreign body into the rectum or has been subjected to anal sex. Careful examination, often under general anesthesia, is required to assess the extent of damage.

Facial trauma or perhaps just a severe nosebleed can result in enough blood being swallowed to cause hematemesis or melena.

Traumatic hemobilia is a rare cause of severe gastrointestinal bleeding. The clinical picture usually begins 7 to 10 days after closed upper abdominal trauma has produced an intraparenchymal hepatic laceration. When the resultant hematoma and liver secretions accumulate within the liver substance, they drain in time through the biliary tree, into the duodenum, producing the clinical picture of an upper gastrointestinal hemorrhage. Eventually the flow slows, the blood in the liver and the biliary tree clots, and biliary obstruction is produced. This results in biliary colic and obstructive jaundice. After another day or so, the whole blood clot passes, sometimes in the recognizable form of the biliary tree, thus relieving the obstruction. Hence, another episode of hemorrhage occurs along with relief of the colic and jaundice. This cycle repeats a number of times until spontaneous healing occurs or surgical intervention becomes necessary.

Traumatic hemobilia is not a difficult diagnosis to reach if an adequate history is obtained and presentation is typical. However, atypical presentations and the rarity of the condition itself both obscure the diagnosis, delaying it in many instances.

The Mallory-Weiss syndrome, in which a mucosal tear at the gastroesophageal junction results from violent vomiting, is rare in children but has been described. Excessive amounts of blood vomited shortly after a previous but violent bout of vomiting suggests the diagnosis, and referral for endoscopic evaluation should be considered.

Intestinal Strangulation

Volvulus or hernial incarceration both cause obstruction to venous outflow initially, which, if untreated, progresses to a venous infarction. During the process, blood oozes into the lumen from the grossly congested mucous membrane, in a similar fashion to blood oozing into the colon from a hyperemic intussusception. Hence, if the volvulus or the hernia is reduced before the stage of infarction, the blood in the lumen of the hitherto closed segment will then be passed through the rectum. Consequently, the passage of blood after an episode of intermittent abdominal pain should alert the physician to the possibility of intestinal strangulation.

Inflammatory Disease

The bloody diarrheal stools of some episodes of gastroenteritis suggest a bacterial etiology, although cultures are required to establish that fact. The blood has important diagnostic significance and implies the need at least to consider intussusception. Hence, if cramps have played a prominent part in the history or if the diarrhea and the general state of the child do not both respond rapidly to aggressive treatment for gastroenteritis, consideration should be given to surgical consultation and contrast radiography.

Inflammatory bowel disease, whether ulcerative or granulomatous, can occur with bloody diarrhea. Granulomatous enteritis is basically a submucosal process, and ulceration with bleeding is a fairly late manifestation. However, ulcerative colitis is primarily a mucosal lesion, and bleeding can be early and sometimes massive. In these conditions, there is usually a long history of cramps, diarrhea, and systemic illness to direct one's attention to pre-existing inflammatory disease. Only rarely is the bleeding so massive that emergency colectomy becomes necessary.

In the hemolytic-uremic syndrome, bloody diarrhea is often a major presenting symptom. The associated hemolytic process and developing renal failure make the diagnosis clear.

Anorectal Lesions

Bleeding from acute anal erosions, or anal fissures, is very common and is diagnosed from the history of blood on the toilet tissue and on inspection of the anus while retracting the buttocks. Gentle retraction of the anus itself will permit visualization even of fissures that are primarily in the anal canal.

Acute diaper rash with perineal erosion and marked excoriation can cause blood on the diaper and can simulate rectal bleeding. Although perineal excoriation is likely to be part of a diffuse diaper rash, careful consideration should be given to the possibility of anal abuse, particularly if the reaction seems to be localized around the anus.

Rare Causes

Several other rare causes of massive intestinal hemorrhage, such as intestinal duplications or arteriovenous malformations, are diagnosed at operation only with few exceptions. The primary physician needs to be aware of them only to include them in the list of differential diagnoses for children going to surgery undiagnosed.

Insignificant Coffee-Ground Vomitus

Some flecks of changed blood, often similar in appearance to coffee grounds, are frequently seen in vomitus if the vomiting has been persistent and over a few days. Many infants being assessed for hypertrophic pyloric stenosis produce "coffee ground" vomitus. Older children with violent vomiting from gastritis or early gastroenteritis may also have traces of red blood or "coffee grounds." These all need to be taken in context since there is little risk of any real significance to "bleeding" of this nature.

Abdominal Trauma

General Considerations

Closed injury of an abdominal viscus is common either as an isolated lesion or as only one component of the multiple injury complex. The effects of closed trauma restricted to the abdomen generally follow recognized patterns, and management is usually quite straightforward. On the other hand, when there are a number of associated injuries, the initial recognition that there is an intra-abdominal injury, the identification of the organ diagnosis, and the selection of the appropriate therapy for the abdominal injury can be extremely difficult. Although most abdominal visceral injuries involve solid organs—liver, spleen, kidney, or pancreas—the hollow viscera are ruptured often enough that one must remain alert to this possibility.

The majority of abdominal injuries in children are caused by closed or blunt trauma. Penetrating trauma, as a result of sharp object impalement or penetration by projectiles such as bullets, is very uncommon in the pediatric age group except in jurisdictions where crimes of violence are particularly prevalent.

Children suffer abdominal injuries when they are struck by hard objects, such as the end of a hockey stick or the center post of bicycle handlebars, or when they fall from trees or apartment windows. Children suffer severe abdominal trauma when struck by moving vehicles, although in this situation multiple injuries are the rule. A child may even sustain organ rupture from compression by the lap-belt portion of a vehicle restraint system, although in most instances this will be preferable to the frequently critical or fatal injuries caused by ejection.

Vehicular accidents, injuring passengers and pedestrians, constitute the single most important cause of multiple trauma during childhood. For every child who is severely injured by a fall from a fifth-floor window or when caught in farm machinery, there are five or 10 children badly injured in road accidents. The injuries sustained by the child pedestrian demonstrate a surprisingly consistent pattern. These observations are discussed in Chapter 44.

Child abuse is an important causative factor in the incidence of abdominal injury. It should always be under special consideration when major abdominal trauma is sustained by a baby. An important clue to a nonaccidental cause for a major abdominal injury in an infant would be the history that it had been caused by "falling from the change table" or some other equally innocuous incident.

Specific Results of Abdominal Trauma

Within the abdomen, the usual effect of closed trauma is laceration of a solid organ resulting in intra-abdominal hemorrhage. The bleeding may be minimal and productive of some pain but no systemic effect or massive and leading to early shock and a fatal outcome. When a hollow viscus is perforated, the result is peritonitis. Therefore, careful assessment of the injured abdomen hinges on the search for signs of continuing hemorrhage or progressive peritonitis.

An additional intra-abdominal effect of closed trauma particularly characteristic of the child is acute gastric dilation. Although one might expect this with a significant abdominal injury, it also occurs frequently with minimal trauma. Gastric dilation following relatively minor trauma often misleads the physician into believing a serious injury is present, a misconception that will persist until effective nasogastric suction has been established.

Hemorrhagic Shock from Abdominal Trauma

Of the potentially correctable mechanisms by which early death results from childhood trauma, massive intra-abdominal hemorrhage may be considered the most common. For this reason, the early detection of continuing hemorrhage is the main focus of repeated examination of the child following abdominal trauma.

Observation following abdominal trauma takes into account not only the local findings but also the systemic manifestations of blood loss. However, with the young child, care must be taken not to place too much emphasis on the blood pressure reading. The child's compensatory mechanisms are so effective that there is often little or no change in pulse or blood pressure until at least one-fourth of the normal blood volume has been lost. Especially active vasoconstriction frequently results in pallor and sweating as well as coolness of the extremities before there are significant and recognizable changes in vital signs. Therefore, one should make the assumption that after trauma the recumbent child who is sweaty and pale has probably lost close to one-fourth of the normal blood volume even though pulse and blood pressure readings are within normal limits. Consequently, in order that treatment can be appropriately prompt and sufficiently aggressive, the accurate diagnosis of hypovolemic shock in its early stages must hinge more on the general appearance of the child than on the pulse and blood pressure recordings. Shock due to blood loss remains largely a clinical diagnosis.

Isolated Abdominal Trauma

Solid Organ Injury

Spleen

Injury of the spleen classically results in left upper abdominal pain; pain with deep breathing because of phrenic irritation; unwillingness to move because of peritoneal irritation; and symptoms of generalized blood loss such as lightheadedness, faintness, and anxiety. In addition, unexplained pain in the tip of the left shoulder is a surprisingly consistent indicator of left phrenic irritation by blood, although sometimes the patient must be lying flat or even in a few degrees of Trendelenburg's position for it to be manifest. The severity of these symptoms varies with the extent of the splenic laceration and the amount of blood lost.

Physical examination may reveal a subject who is grunting from effort to splint the diaphragm and who may show systemic signs of hypovolemia, indicating significant blood loss. Tenderness is usually maximal over the spleen, and peritoneal irritation there and elsewhere in the abdomen is indication of extravasated blood. Rectal examination revealing pelvic tenderness is evidence of free blood in the pelvis.

Abdominal radiography did not play a major role in the assessment of abdominal trauma until computed tomography (CT) became readily available. Plain films may show medial displacement of the gastric bubble by an enlarged splenic mass or crenation of the line of the greater curvature because of bleeding into the gastrosplenic omentum. However, neither of these signs is clearly diagnostic. The CT scan may show not only the size and positioning of the splenic tear, but also that the other parenchymal organs are intact.

Four-quadrant abdominal tap, peritoneal lavage, or diagnostic minilaparotomy are all used frequently to good purpose in adult trauma units, where the presence of significant hemorrhage into the abdomen is considered valid indication for immediate surgery. However, in the conscious child these diagnostic tools are rarely of benefit because bleeding into the abdomen in itself is not indication for operation unless it is massive, in which case the diagnosis is clinically obvious. It is now recognized that the spleen's contribution to the child's immune mechanisms is so important that splenectomy should be carried out only as a last resort. It has also been known for decades that the vast majority of children with evidence of a small to moderate amount of bleeding from an injured spleen will do very well if treated nonoperatively. For this reason, the abdominal tap, peritoneal lavage, and minilaparotomy are rarely indicated in pediatric trauma practice. However, these modalities should be considered in the child who is unconscious from a head injury, who shows signs of hypovolemia, but in whom the source of hemorrhage remains in doubt. A peritoneal tap can also be helpful on occasion when, in the presence of stable vital signs, peritonitis is suspected but confirmation is desired before laparotomy is embarked on.

Notwithstanding the above discussion, it is very likely that further dramatic advances in radiographic techniques, some of the early examples of which are now well established, will remove the need for invasive diagnostic maneuvers such as peritoneal lavage or minilaparotomy except in the rarest of situations. Computed tomography now displays organ contusions and lacerations with an accuracy of definition previously inconceivable. These advances are leading to treatment changes because exact demonstration of the organ laceration preoperatively is making much simpler such questions as not only whether the lesion needs to be repaired but also whether it is readily operable and which surgical approach to use.

Although treatment decisions will continue to require experienced surgical judgment, these decisions will more and more be guided by sophisticated three-dimensional pictures of the injured body zone. It is probable that some children who would previously have been operated on immediately will be treated nonoperatively, and in some instances children who would previously have been treated nonoperatively will benefit from being taken straight to the operating room. It can be anticipated that diagnosis and treatment of traumatic abdominal lesions will hinge more and more on newer imaging techniques.

Surgical techniques are not relevant to this discussion. However, it should be mentioned that laparotomy for a ruptured spleen no longer commits the surgeon to splenectomy. Repair of splenic lacerations and excision of fragments partially detached from the organ, with salvage of most or all of the functioning splenic tissue, have been shown to be practicable and must be the surgeon's goal when confronted with an actively bleeding spleen at operation.

Liver

The severity of liver injuries varies from massive parenchymal disruption with tearing of the hepatic veins away from the inferior vena cava to the small surface laceration which quickly stops bleeding and which leaves the surgeon almost regretting the decision to operate. However, when death occurs within an hour or less of abdominal trauma, the usual cause is massive hemorrhage from a ruptured liver, usually involving hepatic veins, the inferior vena cava, or both.

In general, the clinical picture of the lacerated liver is surprisingly analogous to that of an injured spleen but on the other side. Both can produce very mild symptoms and signs, with slight pain and tenderness with or without pain in the respective shoulder tip, and no indication of hypovolemia, and both can cause marked local manifestations in addition to hemorrhagic shock.

For several decades, the risk of massive bleeding from the torn surface of liver as well as the potential for recovery from partial liver resection resulted in a more aggressive approach to actively bleeding liver injuries. Vigorous blood replacement and major liver resection carried out through a large thoracoabdominal approach has produced survivors. A more conservative approach is receiving some favor currently: the surgeon packs off sites of massive hemorrhage that are encountered at operation with the plan of removing these packs at reoperation 2 days later.

Rupture of the extrahepatic biliary system is very rare as an isolated injury but is occasionally reported in association with right hepatic lobar lacerations. For this reason, the bile ducts must be carefully visualized during any operation for hepatic rupture so that primary repair can be carried out.

Pancreas

Unusual as it is in pediatric practice, acute pancreatitis does occur occasionally, and in the list of possible known causes, trauma rates as the most common. Traumatic pancreatitis may be diagnosed at operation carried out for repair of an associated injury or from markedly elevated amylase levels obtained after closed trauma. Although traumatic pancreatitis of mild to moderate severity usually subsides under careful medical support, surgical repair of major lacerations, excision of a devascularized tail or one isolated from the body by a through-and-through laceration, and drainage of a collection of pancreatic secretions are procedures that are necessary from time to time. These lesions are being diagnosed with increasing accuracy with the help of the CT scanner.

An uncommon but important complication of pancreatic injury is the traumatic pseudocyst. This lesion results from encapsulation of a collection of pancreatic exocrine secretions that have escaped from the organ through a laceration. In most instances, there is a history of closed abdominal trauma several weeks prior to the onset of abdominal discomfort, nausea, perhaps vomiting, and discovery of a firm, spherical mass in the epigastrium. The pseudocyst is usually in the lesser sac and so is seen on contrast studies to displace stomach anteriorly and superiorly. The CT scan demonstrates its retrogastric position and its close proximity to the pancreas. Although some pseudocysts resolve spontaneously and others can be treated successfully by percutaneous drainage, the bulk come to surgery. Operative treatment usually consists of anastomosing the cyst to the adjacent posterior wall of the stomach to obtain satisfactory drainage into the gastrointestinal tract and complete resolution of the cyst.

Kidney

Although protected by their retroperitoneal location and by the lower rib cage, kidneys are frequently injured. Microscopic hematuria is the hallmark of minor renal injury and is frequently seen after vigorous contact activities, such as football, even in the absence of specific trauma to the renal area.

Gross hematuria usually signals a more severe renal contusion or laceration and is indication in itself for urgent investigation. The CT scan is very helpful in this situation, readily revealing parenchymal disruption and urinary extravasation. The addition of intravenous contrast medium produces the needed information about renal function. In the absence of a CT scanner, the traditional intravenous pyelogram is still an effective alternative.

Trauma to the renal artery will, on occasion, produce intimal tearing with occlusion of the lumen. The time required for the necessary investigation while making this diagnosis generally precludes successful renal salvage.

The most serious renal injury of all is avulsion of the renal pedicle, which immediately renders the kidney ischemic and produces massive hemorrhage in the retroperitoneum. Aggressive treatment for shock, which is required for survival, will doubtless occupy all management efforts, at least initially, although tamponade of the hematoma within fascial planes may slow blood loss sufficiently to permit some basic investigation. If so, emergency pyelography to establish the presence of one functioning kidney, followed by emergency laparotomy for control of hemorrhage, will be the most likely sequence of events. At operation, the choice of prompt nephrectomy versus vascular repair in the attempt to salvage the kidney depends on the patient's circulatory status, the capability of the operating team, and the time elapsed since the accident.

In general, emergency surgery is rarely required to deal with blood loss from renal trauma because the perirenal fascial tissues contain extravasated blood fairly effectively, in contrast to the free access which blood from spleen or liver has to the peritoneal space. Consequently, when hematuria following trauma points to the kidney as the target organ, there usually is ample time for a careful evaluation of renal function bilaterally.

All renal trauma, even the most minor, requires careful long-term surveillance of both renal function and the subject's blood pressure. Partial ischemia or renal scarring from contusion can cause a form of delayed hypertension that, if detected early, is eminently treatable, either through nephrectomy or rarely through vascular repair.

Hollow Organ Injury

Stomach

Gastric rupture from closed trauma is uncommon and, for practical purposes, is seen only if trauma is sustained when the stomach is distended. Hence, when gastric rupture is encountered at laparotomy for a perforated viscus, careful exploration of the entire peritoneal space is necessary because fragments of ingested food can be found as far away as the pouch of Douglas.

The severe and very acute peritoneal irritation resulting from gastric perforation is comparable to that seen with ulcer perforation in adults. Free intraperitoneal air may accumulate in such large amounts after gastric rupture that the diaphragm can be displaced upward and respirations compromised. This is particularly true in the young infant, in whom emergency abdominal paracentesis may be necessary to relieve the pressure and facilitate respiratory function. This injury is most unusual in infancy as a result of accidental causes. For this reason, child abuse should be kept in mind when a small baby suffers gastric perforation.

Duodenum

Intraperitoneal perforation of the duodenum is rare. The diagnosis is made either at operation or by visualization of swallowed contrast medium as it leaks into the abdomen. Although also uncommon, retroperitoneal perforation is encountered more frequently and may be assumed to be present when bubbles of retroperitoneal air over the right iliopsoas muscle are noted on plain radiographs. Contrast studies will also demonstrate the perforation. Urgent surgical correction is necessary.

Hematomas in the wall of the duodenum can occur after trauma and produce the clinical picture of duodenal or upper small bowel obstruction. Contrast studies are useful and will usually give the diagnosis. Over the years surgical treatment has varied from serosal incision and evacuation of the hematoma to gastroenterostomy to bypass the obstruction. Currently the availability of intravenous hyperalimentation has resulted in a much more conservative surgical approach because it is now believed that the obstruction will gradually subside in most instances.

Small Intestine

Perforations of jejunum or ileum are encountered from time to time. It is important to remember that the clinical signs of perforation can be delayed for as long as several days after the accident. It is recognized that pouting small bowel mucosa can occlude the mural defect and prevent leakage into the peritoneal space until peristalsis resumes. This is only one of the many reasons for continued surveillance of patients who have sustained closed abdominal trauma and who are being treated nonoperatively. Progressive ischemia of bowel may be the result of a mesenteric injury.

Although small bowel injury is the classic seat-belt injury, there have been a variety of injuries caused by the seat-belt, including
1. Linear bruising of the anterior abdominal wall
2. Intestinal perforations, which may not be manifest for several days, or traumatic pancreatitis
3. Unstable lumbar fracture-dislocations
4. Damage to the spinal cord (usually at the L2, L3, or L4 level) or to the cauda equina

Large Intestine

Colonic perforations are rare but require prompt surgical management to prevent serious septic complications.

Bladder and Urethra

The full bladder is particularly susceptible to rupture when it bears the brunt of closed trauma. Following lower abdominal trauma, the physician must look carefully for peritoneal irritation and be ready to assess the bladder with a cystogram, using pre-evacuation and postevacuation films in both anteroposterior and lateral planes.

On the other hand, most cystic and urethral injuries are caused by impalement on a bony fragment from a fractured pelvis. For this reason, particular care must be taken to assess bladder and urethra when pelvic fractures are suspected. With pelvic injuries, one drop of blood at the meatus should be enough to alert the physician to the possibility of urethral damage. In such instances, there must be no attempt to introduce a catheter until urethral integrity has been demonstrated by a retrograde urethrogram.

Penetrating Abdominal Trauma

The principles of evaluation and management of abdominal injuries caused by penetrating trauma are similar in children to those followed in the care of adults. Most require abdominal surgery, and immediate surgical referral is required.

Foreign Body Ingestion

General Considerations

The ingestion of a foreign body must be the most common, or at least is close to being the most common, physical insult to the gastrointestinal tract encountered in early childhood. The list of swallowed objects seen either by radiograph or after being passed includes small toys or parts thereof, jewelry, coins, pins, needles, nails, screws, nuts, bolts, washers, fruit pits, stones, and dirt. Virtually anything small enough to negotiate the oropharynx has been seen either satisfactorily traversing the digestive tract or stopped somewhere en route.

Although most of these cases are examples of babies or toddlers exploring their environment, some are suicidal gestures by teenagers. In such teenagers psychiatric assessment will clearly be needed, and the referral should be made early, when the family and patient are still concerned about the medical aspects of the situation and much more willing to talk openly.

The ingestion of toxic liquids or other harmful absorbable materials is discussed in standard pediatric texts and poison manuals.

History

Unquestionably many ingestions of harmless objects occur without anybody the wiser. However, many such children do appear in emergency departments after known or suspected ingestions. There may be the history of the child putting a small foreign body in the mouth and having a brief choking spell, followed by the realization that the object is missing. Often there is no coughing or choking noted, and the only information obtained is that the small object with which the child was playing now cannot be found.

Children who have swallowed solid objects are usually complete-ly asymptomatic, although the child with a foreign body stuck in the esophagus can frequently point to the level at which it is located. Difficulty in swallowing may be due to an object that is stuck in the esophagus. A foreign body caught in the upper esophagus at the level of the larynx or cricoid may cause hoarseness and coughing due to irritation of the larynx.

Examination

On examination, there is usually nothing of significance to find. There may be an abrasion or small laceration on the palate or elsewhere in the mouth if the object swallowed was sharp or abrasive. There are rarely thoracic findings even if the object was aspirated instead of in-gested. Abdominal examination is generally normal.

Investigation

Radiographic study is required and should include chest and abdo-men. One must establish that an object which is present is indeed in the abdomen and not in the chest. It is also useful to be able to assure a parent that the child suspected of having swallowed a metallic for-eign body has neither ingested nor aspirated it. However, before one can do that, it is necessary to cover by radiograph not only the chest, but also the entire alimentary tract from incisors to anus. Occasional-ly a foreign body is missed on the first study, but when complications arise, further review of the films reveals an end of the object in the pharynx at the extreme upper limit of the chest film. Such an object is rarely missed when there is a proper study including the mouth and pharynx.

Great care must be taken in radiographic interpretation when searching for some kinds of objects. Pieces of eggshell lodged in the pharynx may be missed on the films initially but identified in retrospect when their presence has been proved endoscopically. Coins lodged in the esophagus are usually oriented in the coronal plane, in contrast to the sagittal plane, in which they commonly lie when in the trachea.

Although radiolucent foreign bodies are also ingested from time to time, it is unusual for clinical symptoms to arise from other than metallic foreign bodies, unlike the comparable situation in the chest, in which radiolucent material can result in pulmonary complications as readily as metallic objects, is more difficult to identify or locate, and consequently is frequently treated late.

Management

Most foreign bodies pass through the digestive system readily and with little holdup. Some larger objects tend to be arrested in the esophagus, coins being prime examples of this, although anything which passes through the cardia into the stomach is rarely held up lower down.

If a Foley catheter can be introduced past a foreign body lodged in the esophagus, pulling the catheter back after the bag is partially inflated has been shown to be effective in many instances. This should not be attempted, however, except under strict fluoroscopic monitoring and with airway control immediately at hand. At The Hospital for Sick Children, the paucity of complications from direct endoscopic removal and the sporadic reports, albeit anecdotal in most cases, of aspiration during the catheter method have resulted in our continuing use of endoscopy as the method of choice.

An object that has reached the stomach can be left alone in most instances. Those in significant danger of perforating will need careful follow-up and surgical advice. These objects include open safety pins and straight pins greater than 2 or 3 cms in length. Repeat films to ensure progression of the object are indicated, and surgical referral is needed should a pointed object such as an open safety pin appear to have stopped.

Those subjects followed at home must be instructed to return promptly in the event of any symptoms referable to the gastrointestinal tract.

Complications

Intestinal obstruction is a very unusual outcome of foreign body ingestion. Cases have occurred in which duodenal obstruction has resulted from the ingestion of a number of plum pits, all of which lodged in the duodenum and totally occluded the lumen. Sunflower seeds can cause difficulty if the hard seed shells are swallowed as well. In this instance, the tough shells can accumulate high in the rectum, where they are retained in a hard, inspissated mass that must be broken up under general anesthesia before it can be expelled.

Disk battery ingestion has become relatively common since these sources of electrical energy have been used for watches and other small appliances. In several instances, these have resulted in perforation, probably as a result of electrolytic action on the mucosa. However, it is now believed that the risk of this sort of problem developing is exceedingly small, unless the battery is held up for a prolonged period at one site, such as in a Meckel's diverticulum or at the ileocecal valve. If the battery is shown to be progressing satisfactorily, no therapeutic measures are warranted. It will probably be passed within a few days.

The Chest

Breast Lesions

Adolescent Breast Hypertrophy

Beginning several years or so before puberty, boys will frequently present with a tender enlargement of the small fragment of breast tissue deep to the areola. This is presumed to be hormonal in origin in spite of the fact it is usually one-sided or, when bilateral, has an earlier onset and progresses to a greater degree on one side. Such patients are sometimes seen in the emergency department because the lump so produced may be quite tender. On occasion the tenderness is such that pain is produced when clothes are merely rubbing on the affected breast. The term ''pubertal mastitis'' is often used for this condition, although it is not generally considered to be inflammatory. In addition, any breast lumps generate fears of cancer, even though they may not be voiced. Complete reassurance is justified because this is not cancer and will not become cancer.

Adolescent mammary hypertrophy in the boy is first noted any time from age 11 or 12 on, is self-limited, and usually subsides within 2 years. In the rare instance, the degree of enlargement is such that the young male patient avoids team sports, swimming, and other physical activities because of fear of ridicule by peers. Simple mastectomy done through a circumareolar incision is a procedure that can be done on an ambulatory surgery basis. Although excision is rarely needed, it can be reassuring to an anxious boy to know that there is an effective treatment in the event the organ enlarges to a degree requiring definitive measures.

A similar form of unilateral mammary hypertrophy can occur in the preadolescent female breast. This may also subside within a year or so or may persist until pubertal breast enlargement replaces it. In the female, it may begin as early as age 10 and may result in continuing hypertrophy with the consequence that the fully developed post-pubertal breast may be significantly larger than the other breast. These girls may also have sufficient tenderness early on that they are seen in the emergency department. Full reassurance is warranted. Any surgical approach, should such be considered because of marked asymmetry, must be delayed until after full pubertal breast development has occurred.

Breast Abscess

In the neonate, the normally engorged breast tissue is susceptible to infection, presumably through the nipple, and the bacterial mastitis which results may progress to form an abscess. The usual etiologic agent is *Staphylococcus aureus*, and appropriate antibiotic therapy will result in quick resolution in most instances unless fluctuation has occurred, in which case surgical drainage will be necessary.

For the breast abscesses that are seen occasionally in the pubertal girl, antibiotic therapy is in order, and surgical incision will be needed when suppuration is evident.

Empyema and Pneumatoceles

Empyema

Although thoracic empyema is seen much less frequently now than it was 20 or 30 years ago, it has not disappeared and remains virtually the only surgical complication of pneumonia that has the potential to require emergency treatment.

In the 1950s and early 1960s, acute empyema and pyopneumothorax, often under tension, were serious surgical complications of staphylococcal bronchopneumonia in infancy and early childhood. Any infant with diffuse bronchopneumonia involving one or both lungs was assumed to have staphylococcal pneumonia and to be at high risk for acute tension pyopneumothorax, sometimes bilateral, which required immediate tube thoracostomy. When these tubes were inserted, the thin, watery pus was often noted to spurt out under marked pressure and sometimes even hit the ceiling. Dramatic relief of the severe respiratory distress was usually obtained at once by correcting the mechanical problem producing it. When this treatment, instituted promptly, was combined with aggressive antimicrobial therapy for the parenchymal infection, the outcome was generally excellent. Only when pleural drainage was incomplete or delayed did the exudate thicken or become chronic to the extent that closed tube thoracostomy was not adequate. In these children, rib resection and open drainage became necessary, although more extensive surgery, such as decortication, proved to be needed only rarely.

Today staphylococcal pneumonia and the complications of it are rare because of steady progress in antibiotic management of bacterial infections. However, with further emergence of drug-resistant strains of many organisms and the ease of international travel from less well-developed countries, it is necessary to remain alert to staphylococcal disease and its complications. Except for the tension pneumothorax of trauma, acute tension pyopneumothorax remains almost the only indication for emergency tube thoracostomy in infancy. It would be regrettable for acute staphylococcal empyema to remain unrecognized and untreated merely because it has become very uncommon.

Other bacterial pneumonias, such as those due to pneumococcus, *Streptococcus*, or *Haemophilus influenzae*, can also on occasion develop pleural complications. However, only rarely does the acuteness of onset or severity of the clinical effects require the immediacy of treatment so often needed following staphylococcal pneumonia.

The number of children who are taking immunosuppressive drugs or receiving chemotherapy for malignant disease is steadily increasing as newer and more effective treatment regimens are being used and children who formerly did not survive continue to live. More often the problem is encountered of the immunosuppressed child with pneumonia due to an organism not normally a pathogen. The immunosuppressed child who arrives with a fever needs to be carefully assessed for the source of infection. If pneumonia is shown to be present, pleural complications must be watched for lest urgent drainage be required.

Pneumatoceles

The other complication that staphylococcal pneumonia frequently causes is the intraparenchymal air cyst, or pneumatocele. With destruction of lung tissue by staphylococcal toxins, air leak into the site, and a one-way valve action permitting entrance of air but obstructing ready egress, an expanding air-filled cyst results. This is usually subpleural but may seem to occupy large areas of a segment or lobe on radiograph. The radiographic differentiation of pneumatocele from congenital pulmonary cyst or, if there are many cysts, from cystadenomatoid malformation may be difficult, although computed tomography will be useful in this regard.

Even large pneumatoceles cause surprisingly little respiratory embarrassment, and the vast majority gradually resolve after pneumonia has been successfully treated. Although very few require emergency measures, the potential for massive enlargement is present, and one should remain alert to the possible need for emergency tube cystostomy if the space occupation by one or more pneumatoceles seriously compromises ventilation.

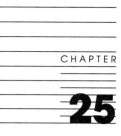
Spontaneous Pneumothorax and Surgical Emphysema

Spontaneous Pneumothorax

Although spontaneous pneumothorax occasionally occurs in the teenager without prior indication of an underlying abnormality, this is distinctly unusual. When spontaneous pneumothorax is encountered, however, the management is similar to that of the adult, with decisions regarding the use of tube thoracostomy hinging mainly on the amount of intrapleural air, its rate of absorption, and the degree of dyspnea created.

Pneumothorax is a recognized complication of asthma, presumably occurring because a peripheral bronchiole has been partially occluded by mucus, thus producing a one-way valve effect. This effect results in overinflation and ultimately rupture of the small subpleural air sac so created. Those physicians experienced in treating asthmatic children customarily look for a pneumothorax, among other complications such as pneumonia or atelectasis, whenever an asthmatic child shows acute deterioration in respiratory function. Few pneumothoraces in asthmatic children progress beyond the stage of a thin rim of air around the lung and rarely require active treatment beyond careful monitoring and treatment of the asthma itself. Preparations should be made, however, for prompt tube thoracostomy in the event of sudden increase in size of the pneumothorax.

Every young adult who carries the late pulmonary stigmas of fibrocystic disease is prone to acute pulmonary crises, any one of which may be due to a pneumothorax. Appropriate treatment in these instances tends to be aggressive because there is always risk of a contralateral pneumothorax also developing unexpectedly. Hence, in fibrocystic patients, any pneumothorax with more than a tiny rim of air around the lung should probably be treated with tube thoracostomy.

Surgical Emphysema

Surgical emphysema is also a fairly common complication of acute asthma, although, unless massive, it rarely has significant physiologic effect. The air may be palpated as subcutaneous crepitus around the base of the neck or visualized in the mediastinum by radiograph, and it may or may not be associated with a pneumothorax. One presumes the interstitial air to be caused by the same mechanism that produces a pneumothorax, although in the case of surgical emphysema, the air manages to dissect centrally along the bronchial tree instead of rupturing distally into the pleural space.

26

Thoracic Trauma

General Considerations

Thoracic trauma is usually seen as part of the multiple trauma complex. For this reason, assessment of the chest, diagnosis of the intrathoracic lesion or lesions, and selection of appropriate management are influenced greatly by the site and extent of other injuries, additional emergency measures that might be necessary, and degree of hemorrhagic shock. One rarely sees a thoracic injury of any degree of severity caused by nonpenetrating trauma that is not associated with other significant lesions.

Closed or blunt trauma is much more common in all age groups than penetrating trauma except in communities where personal assault and street violence are common. Penetrating injuries are rare in the pediatric population. Closed thoracic trauma may be caused by falling from a height or through violence on the athletic field; however, the majority are caused by vehicular accidents.

Although the majority of chest injuries in the older child are accident-related, thoracic trauma in the young infant, particularly in the baby a few weeks old, is likely to be nonaccidental. In the small infant, truly accidental chest trauma of any real significance is very unusual. Child abuse is the likely cause when a small infant is shown to have fractured ribs or any associated intrathoracic damage, whether or not the story of the accident seems valid and consistent with the injuries. In too many small babies, chest trauma presumed to be of accidental origin has been treated by unsuspecting physicians only to have the babies admitted subsequently with additional severe and even fatal injuries.

Rib Fractures and Other Skeletal Injuries

Fractured ribs are seen from time to time and form the hallmark of nonaccidental chest trauma in the small baby, in whom the force is usually a relatively slow manual compression force and frequently causes little or no internal damage. On the other hand, the rib cage in the child appears to be more pliable than it is in the adult, and major intrathoracic damage is often encountered in the child without any evidence of costal fracture. Visible indentations in the chest wall of the young child are sometimes noted after blunt trauma without any radiographic evidence of identifiable rib fractures. This is an example of the same sort of bowing fractures that occur in the forearm from time to time.

Like the adult, the teenager sometimes sustains isolated fractures of one or two ribs from a body-contact sport or a fall without any evidence of pleural or pulmonary complications. These fractures appear in a similar way to those of adults and are treated similarly.

Flail segments of the chest wall due to multiple rib fractures are rarely seen in children, whose ribs tend more to bend than break.

Sternal fractures are rare consequences of anterior thoracic trauma. For practical purposes, these fractures are seen only in older children and are diagnosed and managed in the same way that they are in adult patients. This also applies to another uncommon injury, the sternoclavicular dislocation, in which the medial end of the clavicle dislocates posteriorly or superiorly. This condition can be missed easily on radiographic examination and may require a computed tomographic scan for accurate delineation.

Traumatic Pneumothorax and Hemopneumothorax

Traumatic pneumothorax and hemopneumothorax are typical lesions seen in the older child after closed chest trauma and are almost always situated on the same side as the other apparent injuries. Although the pneumothorax may be stable, quite small in volume, and of little significance, it may enlarge rapidly and can be the cause of severe dyspnea. Traumatic pneumothoraces are frequently under tension and may result in progressive mediastinal displacement, critical compromise of respiratory function, and shock. Although the bone end of a fractured rib may sometimes lacerate the visceral pleura and produce the air leak, this is not common. It is believed that in most instances external compression disrupts lung parenchyma, which then permits air dissection either proximally to cause mediastinal emphysema or distally through the pleura to cause a pneumothorax.

The child who has been hit by a car, who has tire marks on the chest or other indication of closed trauma, and who is grunting or becoming increasingly dyspneic must be assumed to have a pneumothorax or hemopneumothorax that requires immediate drainage. This diagnosis can be made from the foot of the stretcher and requires no sophisticated investigation. Inspection will often reveal the affected hemithorax to be visibly larger than and moving asynchronously with the opposite hemithorax. Auscultation of the chest bilaterally during the few seconds it takes to open the chest tube tray will show decreased breath sounds over the injured side. Tracheal shift may be apparent. Hyperresonance may also be noted but is more difficult to ascertain in the busy and often noisy resuscitation room.

In this situation, tube thoracostomy should be carried out at once. When the local anesthetic agent is infiltrated into the chest wall, the needle can be passed through the pleura and the plunger withdrawn a little. This permits the intrapleural air to be visualized as it bubbles into the syringe through the liquid in the barrel, further confirming the diagnosis. When the tube, either connected to an underwater seal or a one-way valve (Heimlich valve), is unclamped, one can expect rapid lung expansion and almost immediate correction of the dyspnea and the grunting.

When a child is in significant respiratory distress from a traumatic pneumothorax, one should not wait for radiographic confirmation. The diagnosis should be on clinical grounds, and the treatment should be immediate. The purpose of the first radiograph should be to demonstrate the tube in the right place and the pneumothorax eradicated.

If there is an associated head injury, there is even more urgency in the correction of any respiratory embarrassment. A preventable hypoxic episode in the presence of a cerebral contusion can seriously aggravate what brain edema is already present, perhaps leading to untoward sequelae that might otherwise not have occurred.

Current teachings recommend that the tube be inserted in the anterior axilla at roughly the level of the nipple. This site provides excellent drainage for both intrapleural air and blood, and the insertion procedure jeopardizes the heart less than the anterior approach. On the other hand, if an inexperienced physician, singlehandedly responsible for the resuscitation of a child with a traumatic tension pneumothorax, finds the axillary location difficult or awkward, he or she should remember that the anterior location works well too. If drainage does reveal active bleeding, a tube inserted in the anterior location can be supplemented with a second tube laterally in due course.

Although the application of a small amount of suction to the drainage system may speed up lung expansion a little, this is of small significance. The immediate need is to provide drainage of fluid under pressure, and in most instances, the subject's own expirations will rapidly empty the space once the tube is in place.

With few exceptions, tube thoracostomy is not only the resuscitative measure most urgently required, but also the definitive therapy. Relatively few injured chests need to be opened. Even if there is some bleeding from the chest tube, this stops in the majority of cases when the pleural space has been emptied.

In the event of intercostal or major pulmonary laceration, however, bleeding can be active and persistent, sometimes even massive. Few situations can make one feel as ineffectual as when there is massive bleeding through a chest tube without the immediate capability of emergency thoracotomy. In this extreme situation, there is clear and immediate need for massive blood replacement and immediate thoracotomy. This is one instance in which autotransfusion can be lifesaving and can be carried out without the help of a mechanical autotransfuser. Drainage from the chest tube can be collected in a sterile receptacle and immediately reinfused by syringe. We have maintained adequate perfusion pressures through this simple method while bank blood was being obtained and the operating theater readied.

Some experts advocate not draining a large traumatic hemothorax until thoracotomy can be begun, in the hope that the tamponade so created might slow the bleeding. However, for practical purposes, the treatment of choice for traumatic hemopneumothorax remains immediate tube thoracostomy.

Traumatic Asphyxia

Compression trauma to the chest results in a retrograde pressure wave within the valveless jugular venous system. If the pressure is greater than the venules are able to withstand, they rupture, producing multiple petechiae. These are seen over the upper chest, shoulders, arms, and face as well as the oral mucosa, conjunctiva, and retina. Sometimes the myriads of tiny hemorrhages produce a bluish hue to the head and chest, explaining the origin of the term "traumatic asphyxia."

Traumatic asphyxia is seen to some degree in association with many chest injuries and does not alter their treatment. The occasionally quite striking discoloration and the extensive distribution of the petechiae may suggest the possibility of a similar phenomenon inside the skull. Hence, it is somewhat surprising that characteristically traumatic asphyxia has no neurologic effect and when the "rash" subsides there are no sequelae. In some instances, consciousness is obtunded to some degree, although it is difficult to establish that cerebral petechiae are the reason for this instead of hypoxia resulting from the thoracic compression trauma itself.

Other Thoracic Injuries

Traumatic rupture of major airways can produce massive surgical emphysema, which may be restricted to the mediastinum or may spread to the neck, arms and abdomen. There may also be a pneumothorax requiring urgent care. Definitive diagnosis hinges on the distribution of the emphysema, the radiographic findings, and endoscopy.

Injury to major blood vessels causes mediastinal hemorrhage with widening of the mediastinum on the chest film.

Cardiac injuries are rare but should be looked for. Abnormal electrocardiographic findings may be indicative of myocardial contusion.

Cardiac injury with bleeding into the pericardial sac causes progressive cardiac tamponade. When increasing evidence of shock is noted in the absence of a site of major hemorrhage, cardiac tamponade must be considered and pericardial aspiration attempted.

Esophageal perforation from closed trauma is exceedingly rare.

Trauma to the left upper abdomen sometimes causes a traumatic rupture of the diaphragm, resulting in herniation of abdominal contents into the left chest. This is rare on the right side. Traumatic diaphragmatic herniation is a radiographic diagnosis; initial chest films should be examined very carefully for any evidence of herniation, such as location of the gastric air bubble or air-filled loops of bowel above the diaphragm.

Inguinal and
Perineal Lesions

Inguinal Hernia and Hydrocele

Underlying Abnormal Anatomy

Almost all groin hernias in children are congenital (indirect) inguinal hernias. Femoral hernias are most unusual, and the direct or acquired variety of inguinal hernias are rare in pediatric practice.

During fetal development, a peritoneal process or outpouching originating at the internal inguinal ring extends down the inguinal canal, out through the external ring, and, in the male, into the scrotum where it invests the developing testicle. In the female, the process terminates in the labium majus. This peritoneal extension is the processus vaginalis. Except where the process envelops the testicle, its lumen is normally completely obliterated before birth. The portion around the testicle retains its potential lumen and under certain circumstances accumulates fluid, thus forming a scrotal hydrocele, or hydrocele of the tunica vaginalis.

When the lumen of the processus vaginalis fails to become obliterated, one or more of a group of anomalies can arise. If the persistence of the lumen begins at the internal ring where it communicates with the peritoneal space, abdominal contents can protrude down the process, producing an indirect inguinal hernia, the sac for which is formed from the original processus vaginalis. This is a complete hernia if the protrusion extends all the way down into the tunica vaginalis. When the lumen of the processus closes at the internal ring but remains open over a more distal segment, fluid collection in the open portion produces a "hydrocele of the cord." Both a hernia and a hydrocele may be present at the same time, or, alternatively, a hernia can first appear in an older child who had a hydrocele in infancy.

The unknown agent that arrests the process of closure of the processus vaginalis before it has gone to completion may affect both sides; in fact, bilateral hernias or hydroceles are fairly common occurrences. That hernias or hydroceles are more common on the right side probably depends on the fact that obliteration of the lumen of the process is later in going on to completion on the right side than on the left. Hence, it is assumed that the factor which acts to arrest the process prior to completion is more likely to affect the process on the right than that on the left.

The hernial contents in the male child usually consist of small bowel and occasionally omentum. Rarely extraperitoneal portions of colon appear in the hernia, making it a sliding hernia.

A fact frequently not recognized is that the organ most often contained within an indirect inguinal hernia in a baby girl is the ovary. Until a female child has grown to the stage that the abdominopelvic proportions are of adult relationship, the ovary tends to be located just deep to the internal ring and, hence, is considered to be an abnormal organ in infancy.

The relationship between inguinal hernias and undescended testicles is of significance. During fetal development, as the descending testis leaves the abdomen at the internal ring and proceeds down the canal en route to the scrotum it is accompanied by the processus vaginalis. When descent of the testicle is arrested before it reaches the normal intrascrotal position, obliteration of the processus vaginalis is also arrested. Hence, although bowel may not have herniated into the sac, there is always patency of the processus vaginalis and at least a potential hernia associated with every truly undescended testicle (cryptorchid).

On the other hand, the ectopic testicle deviates from the normal descent route and usually ends up outside the external ring in the superficial inguinal pouch. It is not a truly undescended testicle, nor is it often associated with patency of the process or a resultant inguinal hernia.

Clinical Presentation

The diagnosis of inguinal herniation in infancy is often based solely on a clear history from a competent observer such as the child's parent. The presence of a swelling over the external ring or passing down into the scrotum when the baby cries or strains or when the older child coughs is solid evidence for herniation. Confirmation is obtained when reduction occurs under the examiner's eyes or fingers.

When no mass is present at the time of examination, one can attempt to produce herniation by inducing the baby to cry while compressing the upper abdomen, thereby increasing intra-abdominal pressure. While the older child stands and strains down, the examiner can also manually squeeze the abdomen. If these measures do not produce visible herniation, it is unlikely that any maneuver will be successful in doing so. An observation providing additional support for the diagnosis is palpable thickening of the cord on the side of the suspected hernia.

In infants and young children, one should not insert the finger into the external ring to "feel the impulse" with straining, as is customary with adults. The canal can be so short in the young patient and the external and internal rings so wide and almost overlapping that the examiner's finger can virtually enter the abdomen in the absence of any patency of the process. This can lead to a false-positive diagnosis of hernia.

If the history is unequivocal, there is less need to demonstrate the hernia. However, if the history is not clear, attempts to display the herniation and verify the diagnosis are worthwhile.

A hydrocele of the tunica vaginalis appears as a cystic mass in the scrotum, which may obscure the testicle itself. It may be soft and floppy or hard and tense. Although a hydrocele usually transilluminates readily, some scrotal hernias also may transilluminate. The important differential point is one's ability to feel intact cord above the hydrocele. When the scrotal mass consists of herniated intestine, there will be bowel palpable above the mass as part of the cord contents.

When the hydrocele is restricted to the cord, it may ride within the inguinal canal or outside the external ring above the testicle. When in the canal, it is deep to the external oblique muscle and more difficult to palpate in detail. To establish that such a mass is part of the cord contents, one can pull down gently on the gonad and feel the cyst move downward a similar distance, or one can cause the testicle to elevate by pushing upward on the cyst.

Complications

When bowel that is out in an inguinal hernia is pinched off at the external ring so that it cannot be reduced and its lumen is obstructed, the hernia is said to be incarcerated. When a hernia remains incarcerated long enough that the venous return from the herniated bowel, and eventually its arterial inflow as well, begins to be compromised, that hernia is strangulated.

Although the strangulated inguinal hernia is one of the most common causes of small bowel obstruction worldwide, most strangulated hernias in developed countries appear as inguinal lumps that have persisted for a few hours, long before the abdominal cramps, distention, and vomiting of bowel obstruction have developed.

When an inflammatory mass is noted over the external inguinal ring in a baby girl, it is important to remember that the ovary strangulates more often than bowel. The tender, red mass over the external ring which is produced when an ovary strangulates within an inguinal hernia can be confused with an inguinofemoral abscess. However, one should remember that inguinal lymph nodes are situated below the inguinal ligament and are not located within or superficial to the inguinal canal. Furthermore, in baby girls, the absence of the clinical picture of intestinal obstruction should not be taken as evidence that an inguinal mass is not a strangulated hernia, as it might be were bowel strangulated instead of ovary.

Management

The risk of incarceration or strangulation of an inguinal hernia is inversely related to the age of the child. Consequently, inguinal hernias in babies under 1 month of age require urgent repair (within a few days). When an inguinal hernia is diagnosed at birth, repair should probably be carried out before the baby goes home for the first time. With progressively older infants, the degree of urgency decreases; toddlers are customarily scheduled for surgery on an elective basis. However, when a child of any age resides far from medical care, repair of an inguinal hernia is indicated as soon after diagnosis as practicalities permit. Furthermore, because inguinal hernial sacs in general do not close spontaneously, some risk of incarceration always remains. Hence, repair of a hernia should not be put off indefinitely regardless of age.

The presence of an undescended testicle associated with a clinically evident inguinal hernia is reason to delay repair until an age suitable for orchiopexy, provided that the hernia remains readily reducible. However, when the hernia needs repeated and concerted efforts to reduce, combined hernial repair and orchiopexy are indicated on an urgent basis.

When one encounters a baby with an inguinal hernia that does not reduce spontaneously, manual reduction should be carried out before the hernia becomes irreducible. If reduction can be achieved, careful, planned surgical repair can be done on an elective basis, at minimal risk, and with very small incidence of subsequent recurrence. If attempts at manual reduction fail, emergency surgical repair will be required, with significantly greater risk of surgical or anesthetic complication and a higher recurrence rate.

In attempting to reduce an inguinal hernia that has been out for some time, one should not merely apply direct pressure on the mass because doing so will probably result only in flattening out or "pancaking" of the hernia over the upper margin of the external ring. When this occurs, reduction becomes very unlikely. To prevent this pancaking effect, it is necessary to push on the hernial mass from above with the fingers of one hand to keep it from rolling up over the upper margin of the ring, while at the same time squeezing the mass from below with the other hand in a manner similar to the way one squeezes a tube of toothpaste from its lower end. Reduction is usually easy to feel as it happens. Complete reduction is established by feeling empty cord under one's fingers.

Although a hydrocele does not require emergency care or consultation, parents can be very concerned when they see it for the first time. In addition, because hydroceles sometimes appear suddenly and can be tender, urgent advice may be sought. In either situation, it is important to be able to rule out a true emergency and provide the appropriate reassurance. Rarely an acute hydrocele cannot be differentiated from an incarcerated hernia and so may be encountered at operation for presumed hernial incarceration.

When a hernia cannot be reduced by manipulation, immediate surgical exposure, reduction, and repair are indicated. In the past, reduction was often attempted using the method of taxis, in which the child was sedated and positioned head-down in bed for several hours. Although hernias sometimes reduced spontaneously under these conditions, the majority did not, and the operation became necessary several hours later in the course of the disease. Immediate surgery is now recommended when concerted effort to reduce the hernia fails. Tight compression of the hernial contents at the external ring causes testicular infarction as often as bowel infarction, making emergency surgery even more strongly indicated.

Scrotal Lesions

Testicular Torsion

The single serious acute scrotal condition to which one must be constantly alert is torsion of the testis. Too often the definitive treatment of testicular torsion is delayed to the stage of infarction because the diagnosis has been assumed to be epididymitis. In most instances, this can be avoided by remembering to consider torsion whenever an acute scrotal condition is encountered. Torsion can often be eliminated through a careful history taking and examination. However, when doubt remains, prompt surgery and investigation, which not only establishes the diagnosis but also is immediately available, are the only satisfactory alternatives. No child should be treated for epididymitis unless the physician can be certain he does not have testicular torsion.

Testicular torsion can occur in any age, although in neonates it is seen at delivery and rarely in the emergency department. The onset is generally gradual, with a buildup of scrotal pain and soreness over 6 to 12 hours. The "crashing" acute onset frequently described as typical is not seen very often. Although vomiting may occur, it is not a consistent symptom. Systemic symptoms of any sort are unusual.

The child with a testicular torsion will usually arrive on a stretcher; however, a few are able to walk in. In advanced cases, examination reveals a swollen, reddened scrotum with an absent or markedly decreased cremasteric response. The testis will probably appear to be positioned higher than normal. Diffuse tenderness will be noted, and one will not be able to identify one area on the gonad that is more tender than the rest. In such a classic case, the diagnosis of torsion should be made; immediate referral for surgery is necessary.

In the early stages, both symptoms and signs will be proportionately less marked, and the diagnosis will be more difficult to confirm.

A pertechnetate nuclear scan of the scrotum is of greatest value and can distinguish between ischemia of the testis and a normal blood supply. A Doppler arterial reading over the body of the testis has been recommended but is less dependable than the nuclear scan in identifying the ischemia of torsion.

Testicular torsion requires immediate surgery to attempt to salvage the gonad. Unfortunately, when the clinical picture is such that the diagnosis is simple and straightforward, the testis is likely to be irretrievably compromised, and removal may be the only recourse. When the diagnosis is less definite, immediate exploration is even more important because there may still be a chance of testicular survival. Hence, a nuclear scan carried out to make the differentiation from inflammation can be justified only if it can be carried out without significantly delaying the operation, which must immediately follow if torsion is demonstrated. If logistical factors do not permit completing the scan without delaying the operation, taking the child directly to the operating room is warranted. In this situation a surgeon need never apologize for exploring a scrotum in which epididymitis is discovered. Little or no harm is done to the inflamed gonad by the procedure, and the risk of leaving a twisted testis in situ is never worth taking.

The twist in the spermatic cord in almost all instances occurs within the tunica vaginalis. There is a predisposition to twist because the attachment of the epididymis and testis to the tunica is limited to an abnormally small area of the site of entrance of the cord. This pre-existing abnormality is the "bell-clapper" deformity and is in contrast to the normal situation, in which the gonadal attachment is along several centimeters of the length of the epididymis, thus preventing torsion. The bell-clapper deformity is bilateral in most instances, so that when torsion of one testis occurs, the bell-clapper deformity must be assumed to be present also on the opposite side. Fixation of the contralateral gonad should be carried out either during the initial operation for torsion or later on a planned, elective basis.

Torsion of an undescended testicle should be considered when a tender inguinal mass occurs in association with an empty hemiscrotum. Similarly, torsion of an abdominal testis is a good possibility when ill-defined abdominal pain and indefinite signs occur in a boy whose scrotum is empty on the side of the predominant symptoms.

Torsion of an Appendix Testis

In many male children, attached to the upper pole of the testis or adjacent epididymis is a soft tag of tissue up to 4 or 5 mm in length and connected to the gonad or epididymis by a narrow, stringlike attachment that is prone to twist. Such appendages of the testis are embryonic remnants of the müllerian duct system.

As it does in most sites, torsion produces initial obstruction to venous drainage. This causes marked engorgement of the appendiceal tissue before arterial inflow ceases. The result is a tender nodule over the upper pole of the testicle that may be as large as 1 cm in diameter.

The clinical picture of torsion of an appendix testis varies from a small, mildly tender nodule, which is only of minor nuisance value, to the much less frequent large, very tender mass simulating testicular torsion. In most instances, careful and gentle examination reveals a testis that is not elevated, displays a normal cremasteric reflex, and is not particularly tender over most of its substance. However, there will be tenderness at the upper pole, where an identifiable, firm, tender nodule can often be clearly felt. If illumination is satisfactory, one can sometimes see the dark, blue-black nodule move as the testicle moves. This is the so-called blue-dot sign. Rarely there is enough extravasation of blood from the surface of the engorged appendage into the tunica vaginalis that there is marked tenderness and the appearance of diffuse enlargement of the entire testis. In such unusual instances, differentiation from torsion of the gonad itself becomes very difficult without specialized investigative procedures such as a nuclear scan.

Torsion of an appendage does not cause systemic symptoms.

Idiopathic Scrotal Edema

Although idiopathic scrotal edema is relatively uncommon, it can mimic an intrascrotal catastrophe to the extent that immediate surgery seems indicated. Many surgeons confronted with this condition for the first time have proceeded with surgical exploration on the basis that torsion cannot be excluded.

The child with idiopathic scrotal edema will usually have a history of a day or so of scrotal discomfort before seeking medical help. The degree of pain is rarely severe, and the child will probably walk into the department with little evidence of even a protective gait.

On examination, one side of the scrotum will be reddened and enlarged and may have the appearance of an acute scrotal catastrophe. However, careful inspection will demonstrate the normal scrotal rugae to be partially obliterated with edema, and gentle palpation will reveal the enlargement to be caused by edema restricted to the scrotal wall. The gonad can usually be palpated satisfactorily enough to show it to be quite mobile, nontender, and of normal size.

At this stage the examiner will frequently realize that the edema is also present superior to the scrotum, up to and over the inguinal canal. Inspection may also show edema in the perineum behind the scrotum along the one side of the midline and extending as far as the anus. Idiopathic scrotal edema may be bilateral, although when involving both sides it is usually much more marked on one.

Several theories have been postulated, but the etiology of this condition remains in doubt. For this reason, no logical, cause-related treatment is recommended. On the other hand, the condition subsides within a few days, and there are no known sequelae.

When the diagnosis is clear, scrotal edema does not require admission, although restricted activity or even bed rest for a day or two may speed resolution. When the diagnosis is unclear, admission, consultation, or both are warranted to exclude more serious conditions, such as testicular torsion.

The importance of idiopathic scrotal edema lies in the need to be aware of it so that unnecessary surgery can be avoided.

Epididymitis and Orchitis

When asked how to treat epididymitis in a child, many experts in the field will say "you treat epididymitis in the child by operating on his torsion." The very pointed inference to be drawn here refers to the relative infrequency of epididymitis in children as compared with emergencies requiring immediate surgical care. Too often a boy is received whose testis is necrotic because torsion has remained undiagnosed while under treatment for epididymitis.

It should not be unexpected for epididymitis to occur as a complication of a severe and clinically evident urinary tract infection, gonococcal urethritis or prostatitis, lower urinary tract tuberculosis, or congenital syphilis. Ascending infection and epididymitis may also occur after an indwelling catheter has been in place for some days or after some other form of instrumentation. However, in the absence of a situation clearly predisposing to epididymitis, the physician should be loath to accept it as the diagnosis without another opinion or support provided by a testicular scan. If any doubt still remains, it is better to explore a scrotum with epididymitis than to temporize while a twisted testicle slowly dies.

In the absence of a history of urethral manipulation or a predisposing infection, features that favor epididymitis are fever, lessening of the discomfort with elevation of the gonad (Prehn's sign), and evidence on palpation that the swelling and tenderness are restricted to or much worse over the epididymis itself.

When a specific predisposing infection is known to be present, the choice of antibiotic should be straightforward. Otherwise, broad-spectrum antibiotic therapy appropriate for the common enteric organisms is indicated. Customary symptomatic therapy, such as bed rest, ice packs, and elevation, is also helpful to a varied degree. In unusual cases or if response to treatment is not as expected, laboratory investigation for tuberculous and syphilitic infections is warranted, although these infections are now very rare in most developed societies. Involvement of the testicle itself in epididymal infections, epididymo-orchitis, probably occurs more often than is recognized and responds in most instances to the usual therapy.

Although mumps orchitis, the most common form of orchitis, is generally restricted to postpubertal boys, other types of inflammation restricted to the gonad itself are occasionally seen in younger boys. These can be viral or bacterial. Very rarely testicular infection leads to abscess formation and drainage is required, although when this ensues one cannot help wondering if the abscess might have arisen from a traumatic hematoma that became infected.

As is the case with epididymitis, the critical aspect of orchitis is the diagnosis. Differentiation from testicular torsion is difficult on clinical grounds alone and, for practical purposes, requires laboratory proof that the blood supply to the gonad is intact.

Penile Lesions

Of the many acquired and congenital conditions affecting the penis, just those relatively few lesions that are encountered with any frequency in a pediatric emergency department are covered in this chapter. Trauma is dealt with in Chapter 31. Of the four conditions covered, the first three are seen in the uncircumcised penis and, circumcision advocates might suggest, result from the lack of a circumcision. The fourth occurs in the circumcised penis, perhaps because of the circumcision.

Phimosis

Phimosis occurs when the opening of the foreskin becomes scarred down sufficiently to obstruct the passage of urine. Although some examples are doubtless due to any of a variety of causes, it is likely that a majority are due to fibrosis arising over time as a result of parents' (possibly even physicians') efforts to retract the foreskin during early infancy when it is naturally and normally adherent to the glans penis.

In the first few weeks of life, attempts made to retract the foreskin easily produce small tears in the edge of the foreskin. Although these heal readily by secondary intention, each episode produces a small amount of fibrosis. When this has occurred a number of times, the amount of fibrotic tissue around the foreskin opening forms a hard ring around the margin, the opening of which decreases in size as the fibrotic tissue contracts.

Although phimosis is a slowly developing condition, from time to time such children are brought to the emergency department because difficulty in voiding or frank inability to pass urine has been first noticed, albeit belatedly. If the obstruction is complete or close to being so, efforts to void produce ballooning of the foreskin as the urine collects inside it around the glans. There will be a tough, scarred ring around what opening does remain, and the fine spray of urine will be indication of the site of the tiny aperture. A distended bladder can often be palpated.

If the obstruction is not complete, the child may find he can void in a warm tub, thus obviating the need for an emergency anesthetic. However, if the child cannot pass urine at all, emergency circumcision or at least a dorsal slit is necessary. This is usually done under general anesthesia; however, some will be willing to proceed with a dorsal slit under local infiltration, with the view to carrying out a formal circumcision electively.

Although upper tract effects of the back pressure are not common, these are always a possibility and should be kept in mind should further urinary symptoms or a urinary infection ensue.

An understanding of the pathogenesis of phimosis is important because most cases can be prevented by intelligent advice delivered to the parents of the newborn boy. They must realize that forcible retraction of the foreskin early in infancy is the usual cause. There should be no attempt to retract the foreskin until separation from the glans has occurred spontaneously.

Paraphimosis

In the uncircumcised toddler, retraction of the foreskin to facilitate washing of the penis is common practice. When the foreskin is inadvertently left in the retracted position, either by the child himself or because his mother has been interrupted during the bathing process, the stage is set for paraphimosis.

The minor degree of circumferential compression exerted by the retracted foreskin causes obstruction to venous drainage from foreskin and glans that increases as both become edematous. Progressive congestion and edema of foreskin and glans make reduction of the paraphimosis increasingly difficult.

Because physicians who have never seen the gross edema of a childhood paraphimosis can readily confuse it with an acute allergic reaction, such children are occasionally treated with antihistamines, thus further delaying proper diagnosis and reduction of the paraphimosis. To prevent tissue damage from persistent venous obstruction, prompt reduction of paraphimosis is necessary. Digital compression of the edematous foreskin while the glans is gradually pressed back through the surrounding foreskin is usually successful. However, because the edematous foreskin can easily roll up around the glans to give only the appearance of complete reduction, one must always be careful to feel the tight ring around the penile corona slip over the glans before one can be assured of reduction. Sometimes reduction of paraphimosis proves to be so difficult that general anesthesia is required. Rarely a surgical dorsal slit is necessary to permit reduction.

While the edema is subsiding after reduction, the child may find it more comfortable to void in a warm tub. Complications are unusual, although erosions in the preputial mucous membrane produced by the vigorous manipulations theoretically predispose to infection, and the parents should be warned to watch for this. The risk of recurrent paraphimosis has traditionally been considered indication for circumcision once the reaction from the initial episode has settled. Perhaps a little parental education would be as effective as circumcision and would certainly spare the child both the operation and any complications arising from it.

Balanitis

Cellulitis of the foreskin, with or without pus retention within the foreskin, is seen fairly often in a pediatric emergency department. In the preantibiotic era, this infection subsided steadily with warm soaks. Cellulitis responds even more rapidly now on appropriate broad-spectrum antibiotics directed toward the usual enteric organisms, which are the infective agents in most instances. Warm soaks are useful adjuncts.

If the foreskin is excessively long and a hygienic state is difficult to maintain or if several bouts of balanitis have already occurred, it is reasonable to recommend elective circumcision. However, in the absence of the above, instructions regarding cleansing should be adequate in preventing further attacks.

Meatal Ulceration

A superficial erosion of the surface of the glans penis at the meatus is a common occurrence in the first few weeks after a newborn is circumcised. The glandular mucosa at the meatus is very sensitive to the friction to which it is exposed after circumcision. Rubbing against the diaper, whether or not there is additional irritation from urine, is often sufficient to cause an erosion.

The parent may complain that the baby cries when he urinates and that there is a drop of blood on the diaper when it is changed. Close inspection reveals the ulceration on the edge of the meatus. This will heal readily with the help of petrolatum dressings held in place by the diaper. The parents should also be instructed to change the baby frequently so as not to leave him for long periods with a wet diaper.

As innocuous as meatal ulcerations are, they tend to recur; repeated erosions, with the resultant fibrosis, can produce a scarred and stenotic meatus that requires a meatotomy. If the meatus is beginning to scar down and there is any evidence of decrease in the urinary stream or straining to void is noticed, prompt referral for consideration of meatotomy is important, before the resistance to flow can have any damaging effects on the rest of the urinary tract.

Anal and Para-Anal Abnormalities

Only the conditions directly involving or situated close to the anus in children are included in this chapter. Trauma is covered in Chapter 31. The many congenital lesions generally seen either in the newborn nursery or in a pediatric surgeon's consulting office are dealt with in volumes on neonatal surgery.

Anal Fissures

Anal fissures are common in all age groups. In babies, they are often seen after the passage of a large or hard stool and, occasionally, in a superficial and acute form after a digital rectal examination. In older children, they are consistently associated with hard, constipated stools.

The symptoms caused by a fissure are anal pain with defecation, bleeding, and constipation. On the other hand, constipation is as important in the causation of a fissure as the fissure is in the tendency toward stool retention and constipation.

Blood from a fissure is bright red and is seen on the surface of the stool and on the toilet tissue. For practical purposes, fissural bleeding in children is never of such a magnitude as to cause anemia.

The presence of constipation, anal pain on defecation, and blood on the paper is tantamount to the diagnosis of fissures, the presence of which is confirmed by inspection. Gently separating the buttocks usually everts the anus sufficiently to reveal any fissures. When this is not successful, fissures can be seen through a test tube inserted into the anus. A very tight sphincter noted on rectal digital examination also suggests the presence of a tender anal fissure.

Fissures are common, perhaps the most common, cause of apparent rectal bleeding. Other differential diagnoses include rectal and colonic polyps, intussusception, Meckel's diverticulum, intestinal duplication, inflammatory bowel disease, and other rarer causes of rectal bleeding. However, fissures are unique in that they produce blood that clearly comes from the anus, cause no systemic symptoms, and are associated with constipation rather than diarrhea.

A great many fissures are acute, are superficial, and heal rapidly and spontaneously. Others are persistent and resist treatment, and their management particularly must address both constipation and the lesions themselves.

Significant constipation requires continuing management by the patient's regular physician because treatment of chronic constipation is a long-term issue and cannot be addressed in one visit to the emergency department. However, one can assure parents that the fissures are a small part of the whole picture and will improve as bowel function responds to treatment.

Some fissures, particularly those which are chronic, may require surgical treatment. This may consist of repeated dilation, cauterization, or excision of the fissure or one of the foregoing combined with internal sphincterotomy. As a result, the management of chronic anal fissures embodies a combined medical-surgical approach.

Para-Anal Abscesses

When one remembers that glands of the anal canal are constantly exposed to heavy bacterial contamination, one cannot help but wonder at the relative infrequency of infection and abscess formation in the area.

When debris or mucus obstructs an already contaminated gland, infection arises and develops into a para-anal abscess. As this progresses, it produces a red, tender mass beside the anus that requires surgical drainage. These abscesses sometimes drain spontaneously, although usually incisional drainage is still needed in the majority of cases to make the drainage opening adequate. Fluctuation is rarely detectable in this site, and drainage is determined on the basis of the red, tender, firm mass, which may be best felt by palpation between a finger in the anal canal and the external fingers. The drainage of most such abscesses requires general anesthesia; in the first few weeks of life, quick incision without anesthesia is an alternative.

Anal Fistula

When a para-anal abscess drains externally, the potential for fistula formation is produced. External drainage of a para-anal abscess that has arisen from infection of an anal gland leads to resolution of the immediate infection. However, it also provides a route for subsequent contamination, suppuration, and drainage. This establishes the anal fistula.

The baby with an anal fistula will have a repeated history of pustule formation beside the anus and subsequent external drainage, followed by apparent resolution of that abscess. Between episodes of suppuration and drainage, there is usually a small visible punctum where the drainage occurred that is pigmented and perhaps slightly retracted because of fibrosis. This marks the cutaneous end of the fistula and is the site of insertion of the probe during fistulotomy.

Anal fistulas persist if untreated and need to be laid open surgically from end to end to permit healing. This is done electively under general anesthesia. Even when the fistula passes around the internal sphincter and complete fistulotomy entails dividing the sphincter, this is indicated and in the pediatric age group does not affect continence.

The physician should be aware of the occurrence of anal fistulas as complications of several intestinal diseases, granulomatous enteritis being the most obvious. Hence, the presence of such a fistula in an older child, particularly when abdominal symptoms are associated, should alert one to this possibility.

Rectal Prolapse

Prolapse of the inner layers of the rectum through the anus is an alarming sight to parents when viewed for the first time. However, unless the prolapse is left unreduced for some time, it has little long-term significance, is usually of nuisance value only, and becomes rare after age 2 or 3. Prolapse of all layers of the bowel wall is much less common and usually related to sphincter paralysis or severe malnutrition.

The only important pre-existing pathology to be excluded is fibrocystic disease, although the reason for this relationship is unclear. Investigation for fibrocystic disease is necessary in any child whose rectum begins to prolapse.

Rectal prolapse is also common in the baby who has spina bifida with paraplegia. Here the lax and patulous anus offers little resistance to the prolapsing bowel and treatment is particularly ineffective, although several surgical procedures have been devised to hold the anus in a partially contracted state.

In the usual case, the reason for the ease of slippage of one layer of bowel wall on the adjacent layer is unknown. However, once prolapse has occurred it tends to happen whenever the baby has a bowel movement, especially if he or she is constipated or tends to strain forcefully with defecation.

Manipulative reduction of the prolapsed bowel is easily accomplished. However, the basic objective of treatment is a decrease in frequency of the episodes of prolapse and, if possible, prevention. This requires, more than anything else, careful adjustment of bowel habit and consistency of stool, matters requiring thorough long-term care by the patient's regular physician or a pediatric consultant.

Although a variety of surgical procedures have been carried out for this condition over the years, the customary treatment now is nonoperative and is based on the observation that prolapses occur less often after the age of 2 and disappear almost completely after the age of 3. After age 3 the anterior curve of the coccyx and distal sacrum has developed and is believed to receive most of the downward pressure of defecation, a force which is not resisted in this way prior to age 3 when the sacrum is still relatively straight.

Perineal Trauma

General Considerations

Trauma to the area of the perineum, including the external genitalia and anus, as well as the buttocks and upper thighs is common and fortunately usually of a minor nature. However, more serious injuries do occur and are always of major concern. Pelvic fractures are typical examples. Although all open fractures of long bones are serious and require sophisticated management, the majority occur as isolated injuries and heal well without complications. On the other hand, fractures of the pelvis signal major forces at work and are often associated with intrapelvic visceral and perineal injury as well as hemorrhagic shock. When a pelvic fracture is open to either external or enteric contamination, it carries a guarded prognosis. Because of the high risk of major sepsis, open pelvic fractures have an overall mortality of close to 50 percent.

When sustained in the perineal or gluteal area, even the most insignificant laceration requires surgical care different from that which would be appropriate for lesions elsewhere. One must assume perineal lacerations to be heavily contaminated with gram-negative enteric organisms and the chance of subsequent infection to be high if closure is by primary suture. For this reason, most perineal lacerations are best treated open, at least initially. Secondary closure, or even delayed primary closure, can be considered if the wounds are large enough to justify it. However, such decisions require sophisticated surgical judgment and experience.

Similarly, when splinters or other foreign objects are removed from the perineal or gluteal area, there is a significant risk of infection arising in the wound. Hence, special measures are required in view of this risk, such as laying the tract open, warm soaks, perhaps antibiotics, and careful monitoring.

Trauma demonstrating the whole spectrum of severity is encountered involving the buttocks and perineum, frequently without any reason to suspect nonaccidental injury. However, one must have a particularly high index of suspicion for abuse, sexual or otherwise, when one encounters a child with injuries to the perineum or the buttocks. Traditionally the buttocks have been a recognized site for punitive or disciplinary trauma, and it is logical that in child abuse generally the buttocks and adjacent areas form a common target. In particular, perineal trauma opens up the whole subject of sexual abuse, to victims of either sex. Psychosocial, legal, and medical aspects all require detailed consideration.

For all these reasons, trauma to the gluteal or perineal areas is indicated for serious concern regarding the validity of the history of the incident, the cause of the injury, the appropriate management, the risk of serious infection, and the overall prognosis. Proper management of perineal trauma also requires a degree of consideration of the patient's modesty and feelings of embarrassment that is rarely needed to the same degree elsewhere.

Trauma to the Scrotum

Scrotal injuries are viewed with great concern by medical and lay personnel alike because of the presence of the gonads. Minor contusions of the scrotum and testicles are encountered from time to time and, although painful, heal rapidly with no sequelae. More serious contusions result in hemorrhage into the involved testis, and occasionally a testis is lacerated or ruptured by the blow. Unless testicular swelling is marked or progresses, blunt trauma to the testicle is indication for conservative management, which includes bed rest, elevation of the scrotum, application of ice packs, and analgesics. However, when the gonad enlarges rapidly, suggesting major hemorrhage into the parenchyma of the organ, exploration under general anesthesia may be warranted to release the pressure inside the tunica albuginea or, when required, to suture a gonadal laceration. Major trauma to the testes is unusual, and no practitioner acquires much experience with the condition. For this reason, such cases deserve consultation.

Rarely major avulsion trauma to the scrotal sac is reported. When encountered, the testicles may be seen to be intact and viable although exposed. Urgent referral is required so that the testicles can be covered with skin as soon as possible. This can be accomplished either by repairing the lacerated scrotum about them, if there is sufficient scrotal skin remaining, or by implanting them deep to the skin of the thigh or groin.

Penile Trauma

Contusions

Contusions of the penis are not seen very often because of the ability of the penis to move out of the way of external trauma. However, when the small child of a certain height urinates standing up at the toilet, his penis just appears over the edge of the bowl. If the toilet seat then inadvertently falls, the penis can be caught between seat and bowl. When this or other comparable incidents cause compression trauma, the result is usually a minor contusion with a little swelling, ecchymosis, and tenderness, and the vast majority will quickly return to normal without complication. However, with more severe trauma, penile contusion can cause urinary obstruction because of urethral edema. In the event of difficulty in urination following penile contusion or the observation of a drop or two of blood at the meatus, urgent referral is needed. To demonstrate urethral integrity, a retrograde urethrogram, carried out very gently, is required, followed by careful catheterization if the urethra is shown to be intact. Suprapubic cystostomy is required if there has been significant urethral damage. Therefore, prompt surgical referral is in order for any cases in which there is anything more than a minor superficial contusion.

Zipper Injury

The "zipper injury" is a common summer injury to the uncircumcised penis. When the small boy is in a hurry to get back outside to play and is not wearing underwear, he can readily catch the foreskin in the zipper of his pants as it is carelessly jerked up.

Once this has happened, one can never unzip the zipper without causing additional damage to the foreskin, so it is necessary to release the tissue in some other manner. If the foreskin is not caught in the sliding hasp, it can be released by cutting across the zipper above or below the point of entrapment and pulling the two sides of the zipper apart. There is a dressmaker's tool that is very effective in forcing a zipper apart without having to cut it first.

However, if the foreskin is trapped in the sliding hasp, separating the two sides of the zipper will not release it, and the tissue will need to be anesthetized using local infiltration. Although infiltrating the prepuce is intimidating to the child at the very least, it is usually easily done because the foreskin is composed of very loose tissue and virtually the whole area can be rendered anesthetic from a single needle placement. Once anesthesia has been obtained, the hasp can be pulled back over the trapped foreskin, thus freeing it. Excision of excessively torn or contused foreskin which can result should then be carried out followed by suture closure. In most instances, the residual damage requires no surgical repair and consists of a combination of minor contusion and several small superficial lacerations, which merely require warm sitz baths for a few days. Follow-up to detect infection in its early stages is necessary because the minor lacerations caused in this way seem prone to infection.

Circumpenile Strangulation

In circumpenile strangulation, whether by string or wire in the older child who is perhaps being abused, or by the hair-tourniquet syndrome in early infancy (see Chapter 9), the most important point in treatment is to ensure that all of the encircling foreign body has been removed. In the event that the circumferential constriction has resulted from a snug surgical dressing, one must not only remove the dressing but also ensure that there is no clotted blood adherent around the site; unless this is removed, it can sometimes maintain the strangulation itself or even obscure a constricting thread left behind from the dressing.

Foreign Bodies

Foreign bodies sometimes need to be removed from the penile urethra. Although the insertion of objects into the urethra is usually the action of a disturbed child or possibly an extreme form of self-exploration, the possibility of abuse must be kept in mind.

Most foreign bodies in the penile urethra are easily palpable within the organ. When extending down within a millimeter or so of the meatus, removal with the use of a fine mosquito hemostat should not be too difficult. However, there must be no blind attempt to grasp an object with forceps if it is more than a very few millimeters from the meatus. Referral for endoscopic removal is required.

Major Penile Trauma

Major penile trauma may be inflicted by machinery, industrial or otherwise, or is sometimes reported as the result of actions on the part of a mentally deranged individual. Such mutilation should also bring to mind the possibility of a form of sexual abuse. Cutaneous lacerations of the penis, fractures of the erectile corpora, and partial or complete amputations are possibilities. Prompt referral is necessary.

Complications of Circumcision

Although circumcision is not as frequently carried out as it once was, it is still the most common procedure by which surgical trauma is inflicted on the penis. Undesirable complications following a carefully done circumcision are most unusual. However, hemorrhage, infection of the surgical site, meatal ulcer, separation of the mucocutaneous junction, and partial or complete amputation of the glans are all encountered from time to time.

Postoperative Hemorrhage

Postoperative hemorrhage is usually an extension of operative hemorrhage because what bleeds after the operation is almost always the same vessel that was bleeding during the operation. Although oozing after circumcision is almost always merely a nuisance problem that clears spontaneously, one hears occasionally of the infant who was allowed to bleed into shock unnoticed in the hours after a surgical circumcision. Good operative hemostasis should prevent this situation from occurring, and when it does occur, careful postoperative observation should prevent it from getting out of hand. Attempts to stanch postoperative bleeding by pressure dressing usually fail because of the practical difficulties inherent in trying to apply circumferential pressure to the end of the penis. In most instances, the proper treatment is for the surgeon to return the child to the operating theater and insert stitches where they are needed to obtain hemostasis. It should be remembered that persistent bleeding from a circumcision is a common way for a bleeding diathesis to become manifest in the young infant.

Wound Infections

Minor wound infections are common after circumcision. The site of anastomosis between the glandular mucosa and the skin around the shaft frequently reveals some exudate after the first postoperative day or two. This superficial infection is common and rarely of importance. Occasionally a more severe and spreading infection results and produces acute cellulitis of the penis.

Although the mild, common form subsides rapidly with warm soaks, antibiotic therapy is warranted if inflammation involves the shaft. In the more severe cellulitic form, high doses of antibiotic are indicated. Such infections are usually due to *Staphylococcus aureus* or hemolytic streptococci, although coverage for enteric organisms is also recommended.

Meatal Ulceration

Meatal ulceration is also a complication of the surgical trauma of circumcision. It is discussed in Chapter 29.

Separation of Mucocutaneous Anastomosis

Separation of mucocutaneous anastomosis occasionally occurs after circumcision. This may occur when a crushing clamp or plastic bell has been used or after a ritual circumcision in which the foreskin is pulled forward and amputated without any particular steps taken to make mucosa adherent to skin. Separation does not occur when the anastomosis is properly sutured. Although parents can be reassured of a good outcome provided the separation does not encircle most of the penis, ideally the baby should be seen by the operating surgeon.

Excision of Glans

Excision of part or all of the glans is reported sporadically, usually following a method of circumcision in which the foreskin is pulled forward beyond the glans and then amputated without the glans being under direct vision. When a small and superficial piece of glans distant from the meatus is shaved off, prompt healing can be expected. If the meatus is involved, consultation is required so that measures can be taken to avoid a meatal stricture. If almost the entire glans is excised, little can be done beyond promoting satisfactory healing of the wound. If even a small portion of the glans remains, it may enlarge during growth, especially at puberty, to provide some of the function of the glans.

Straddle Injuries

Slipping forward off the bicycle seat onto the crossbar or falling while walking the balance beam are typical causes of straddle injury to the perineum.

When a boy has sustained a straddle injury, contusions or, less often, lacerations of the urethra are the most common important lesions encountered. The absence of hematuria and the ability to urinate without difficulty are assurance against laceration. However, urethral or periurethral contusion may not be manifest until some hours after the injury when developing edema may result in partial or complete occlusion of the urethra. If increasing difficulty in voiding is encountered some hours post-trauma, consultation and detailed assessment of the urethra is urgently needed to determine the nature and degree of the obstructing lesion. The choice between urethral instrumentation and urinary diversion is much more easily made when some lumen remains.

Rectal digital examination is a basic requirement for proper primary assessment for urethra injury. When the urethra is divided by blunt trauma against the pubic arch, the prostate often rides higher than it does normally and is quite mobile.

If blood appears at the meatus, whether the child is voiding satisfactorily or not, laceration of the urethra must be suspected and careful retrograde urethrography is required before any other urethral manipulation should be permitted. The absence of blood at the meatus does not exclude laceration. Hence, urinary symptoms of any sort following blunt trauma to the perineum require careful urologic assessment.

When a girl experiences a straddle injury, a different approach is required. In this situation, there is risk of both lower urinary damage and damage to the vaginal introitus, and if there is any blood on the perineum, the labia majora should be gently retracted and the introitus inspected in an attempt to determine the source.

The most common lesion to be encountered is a superficial mucosal laceration of a minor labium or of the fourchette posteriorly.

These heal rapidly and uneventfully with cleansing soaks and good hygiene. However, it is crucial to confirm that the blood is coming from the lesions visible on the perineum and not from the vagina. If a moist swab can be inserted into the vagina and removed free of blood, one can be reasonably certain that there is no vaginal source of the bleeding. However, if doubt remains, immediate gynecologic referral with a view to consideration of examination under anesthesia is warranted.

Urethral damage is less likely in girls than is the case with boys. However, hematuria is the prime warning sign of possible urethral damage and warrants careful assessment of urethral integrity before any instrumentation such as catheterization is attempted.

Sexual Assault

In this section the overall management of the sexual assault situation is not discussed in detail. Monographs on the social, legal, and psychological aspects of sexual abuse, which is really one form of child abuse generally, are available. The specimens needed to satisfy evidentiary requirements, the time intervals after which the specimens are of little value, and the need for postcoital prophylaxis against either pregnancy or venereal disease are all covered in detail in sexual abuse protocols or specific advisories and are not mentioned further here. This section does not include a discussion of the psychological injuries sustained by the victims of sexual assault, injuries which so often have longer lasting effects and the sequelae of which are generally more disabling by far than the physical evidence of trauma, which itself may be almost indiscernible.

Physical injuries inflicted by perpetrators of sexual abuse are of many varieties and are seen in many body regions. Although attempted forced intercourse, whether vaginal, anal, or oral, is the form of sexual abuse that comes to mind most often, bruises from pinching or biting or cigarette burns on the breasts or perineum are just a few of the other manifestations. Penile injury from direct violence or the result of elastic band or string constriction are much rarer manifestations of sexual assault, although whenever these or similar injuries are encountered the possibility of sexual assault must always be seriously considered.

The effects of forced vaginal penetration range from perineal tears, sometimes running posteriorly to or into the anus, lacerations restricted to the vagina itself, or minor tears involving the introitus or hymen. The management of such lacerations will vary from layered perineal repair in the formal operating theater for the most severe to warm baths and hygienic measures for the superficial abrasions. As is the case with perineal trauma generally, bleeding from the vagina following forced penetration requires careful and detailed gynecologic evaluation. If significant vaginal bleeding is evident, it is likely that examination under anesthesia will be required to assess the extent of injuries, unless the patient is a sexually active teenager who might allow an adequate vaginal assessment.

When the history reveals forced vaginal insertion of a solid object, serious perineal and intrapelvic damage must be assumed. Surgical management is likely to require both laparotomy and perineal exposure.

Anal penetration rarely causes injury that requires specific therapy, although an acute fissure would be expected. In such instances, efforts directed toward maintaining the stools in a soft state and warm baths should hasten complete healing.

Jennifer Blake, M.D.

Gynecologic Emergencies

Examination and Instrumentation

Few examinations cause as much anxiety to the physician, the family, and sometimes the patient as the gynecologic examination of the young girl. If the physician is not relaxed and confident, it is certain that no one else will be. It is always easiest to learn the basic technique in a nonemergency setting by working with an experienced pediatrician or gynecologist. This enables one to learn an approach that is most comfortable for examiner and patient and gives some familiarity with the wide range of normal anatomy that may be encountered. In the gynecologic examination the guiding principle is: "Above all do not harm." In other assessments and procedures, it is occasionally necessary to restrain a child. With the gynecologic examination, restraint may rarely be necessary with an infant. However, the older child must *never* be restrained because she may recall the event as a sexual assault, and it can give rise to difficulties long after. The following guidelines aid in the approach to the child with a gynecologic injury or complaint.

The Setting

Privacy, quiet, and comfort are essential to a successful examination. If there are personnel bustling in and out, other children popping up from behind privacy curtains, and the sounds of frightened or crying patients filling the air, one is lucky to obtain a history, never mind a physical assessment. It is better to move the child to a more appropriate setting or wait for a suitable room.

Parental Presence

A calm, confident parent can be a great help with some small children, but an anxious parent can ruin all the careful work of the most skilled clinician. The decision is a judgment call, which one should make after observing the interaction between parent and child during the interview. If both parent and child seem highly anxious, remember that an upset parent is unlikely to be able to calm a frightened child and that there will be two patients to deal with instead of one. In this situation, the parent(s) should be asked to wait outside before the physical examination is begun. One then hopes to be able to settle the child before progressing to the gynecologic examination. With teenagers, the parents should not be present so that the teen will have the opportunity to speak freely. It is important for children of any age to have some time alone with the physician. Children may then disclose details of sexual experience that they could not discuss in front of their parents.

Equipment

To visualize the vagina and cervix necessitates the use of a vaginoscope or, in teenagers, a slender speculum (Fig. 32–1). These instruments in inexperienced hands can cause pain and injury. Therefore, during the general examination of the child, the need for internal ex-

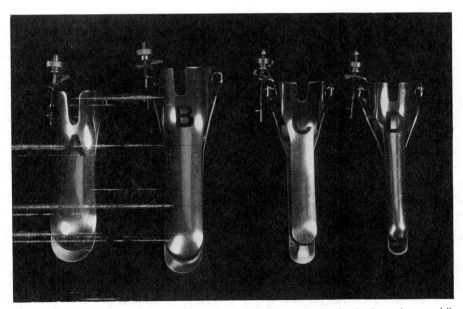

Figure 32–1 *A*, A medium Graves speculum is suitable for patients who have borne children. *B*, This speculum may be used in sexually active teenagers. A narrow Pedersen (*C*) or Huffman (*D*) speculum is suitable for young teenagers.

amination must be assessed. If such proves to be necessary and one has little or no experience in the procedure, arrangements should be made to obtain a clinician who is skilled in the pediatric gynecologic examination. On the other hand, a great deal of information can be gained from a careful external examination. Some basic equipment for this will help greatly and should all be in place beforehand, including

1. An excellent light source
2. Warm saline for irrigation on an intravenous pole with tubing
3. Bags of chilled solution for compresses
4. Saline moistened urethral swabs for vaginal cultures (if needed) and culture media
5. A hand lens or magnifying glasses
6. Lidocaine (Xylocaine) jelly
7. A hand mirror (for the child to watch the examiner or to distract herself)
8. A soft toy for the child to hold
9. A sexual assault kit

The sexual assault kit should always be available. The physician using it should be completely familiar with its contents and must know how to collect evidence that will stand up in court. The assessment for suspected child abuse falls into a category of its own and is best left to a specialized team, the members of which have the skills to conduct the crucial initial history and examine a traumatized child. If such a team is not available, it is important to study the kit carefully beforehand and be gentle and painstakingly thorough.

The Examination

A more productive and generally better gynecologic assessment is performed if it is included as a part of the general examination. This allows the physician some time to get to know the child and the child to know the physician. One should be looking for clues that will help to assess the stage of pubertal development as well as endocrine status. The presence of skin rashes or evidence of infestations should be noted, in addition to the presence of bruising or signs of recent trauma to the kidneys or abdomen. Throughout the examination one first describes clearly and simply what is about to be done and then does what was described and nothing else.

The external genitalia can be examined most easily with the child in a froglike position, in which flexion of the knees as well as flexion and external rotation of the hips readily exposes the perineum. Teenagers and older girls can use lithotomy stirrups. The labia and perineum should be carefully inspected for foreign substances, trauma, or skin conditions. The vaginal orifice can be seen by gently pressing the labial pads downward and laterally or by using a light pulling motion. The child can often help, using her fingers to separate the labia. Most inexperienced observers are surprised by how bright red the tissues appear in childhood. This is a result of low estrogen levels, so that the vaginal lining is not a stratified squamous epithelium but a very thin layer through which the underlying blood vessels can be seen. This surface is extremely sensitive to any sort of insult and subject to minor infection and irritation. The hymen itself can be readily seen at this examination, and a hand lens or magnifying glasses will help detect any breaks or trauma to this tissue. It is crucial to note even minor trauma to the hymen because it may be associated with a far more significant lesion in the vagina or rectum and will necessitate further examination or even examination under anesthesia. Finally, the anus should be inspected for evidence of scratching, suggesting pinworms, or trauma. A patulous anus is suggestive of abuse. A careful rectal examination will enable assessment of the internal genitalia.

Obtaining Cultures

If cultures need to be obtained in a teenager, a proper speculum examination using a slender speculum is essential to visualize the cervix and get a reliable sample. In young girls, because of the immature lining of the vagina, adequate samples can be obtained by collecting vaginal irrigant or by the *careful* use of a saline-moistened swab. A dry cotton swab should *never* be used on a young child because it will tear the fragile tissue. One can see well by depressing the perineum to cause vaginal opening, then, without touching the hymen, the samples can be collected.

Patient Confidentiality

There is an inevitable conflict between the patient's right to confidentiality and the parents' wish to be informed fully of all matters relevant to their child. Statutory guidelines vary as to the age at which parental consent is required and the settings in which it is mandatory. In general, when a child is to be admitted to the hospital or is to undergo an operative procedure, parental consent must be obtained. The patient's right to confidentiality is also protected, and every minor has a right to make an informed choice and give or refuse consent according to her ability to understand the issues at stake. The obligation of the physician is to ensure that the patient is fully informed and participates in the decision making to the extent possible. Issues of disclosure are more complex, but in general protection of a patient's confidences is in her best interest regardless of her age. The absence of free choice may mitigate the duty to protect confidences. If a 15-year-old has chosen to become sexually active, that confidence should be protected. If she is being exploited or sexually abused, she is in need of protection. These judgments require a more extensive history than can be readily obtained in a hospital emergency department. It is a wiser course to involve the adolescent service or social worker with the patient to determine what will be in her best interest. The greatest obstacle to teenagers seeking medical care is their fear of confidences being violated. We would do well to respect them except in extraordinary circumstances.

Trauma

Straddle injuries are the most common source of trauma to the genitalia of a young girl and have a seasonal peak when bicycles come out in the spring. The majority of these lesions involve the labia. Penetrating injuries can cause major intra-abdominal damage, with minimal external findings. Sexual assault must always be considered.

The first step is a general assessment, including an assessment of vital signs, a careful examination for evidence of trauma to other parts of the body, and an abdominal examination. If the child is frightened and in pain, it may be difficult to do a satisfactory gynecologic examination. An ice pack, chilled bag of intravenous solution, or cool compress may be applied and the child allowed to rest quietly for 20 minutes before being reassessed. This may be repeated with a change of compress and will allow a much more useful examination to be conducted.

Before starting, all equipment should be ready. It is most important to be able to visualize the vaginal opening to exclude penetrating injury, and this, as described previously, requires that the tissues be manipulated. To reduce the discomfort in the traumatized area, lidocaine jelly can be applied and left in place for a few minutes to numb the perineal tissues. If old blood obscures the view at the start of the examination, a gentle stream of irrigant set up on an intravenous pole will facilitate inspection of the affected area. Blood from a periurethral tear often accumulates in the vagina and can simulate vaginal bleeding. In the absence of a hymenal injury, the irrigant may help to sort out whether the blood is arising from the vagina or is entrapped old blood.

Small labial hematomas can generally be managed conservatively with ice packs and pressure dressings. Enlarging hematomas require referral to a gynecologist for management.

Lacerations that are not deep and are not associated with any hymenal injury or vaginal bleeding can often be managed conservatively with sitz baths and simple dressings. More extensive injuries require referral to a gynecologist for examination under anesthesia.

In any case of trauma, it is imperative that damage to the rectum or urinary tract be excluded. Abdominal examination and a digital rectal examination should detect gastrointestinal injury. After the genitalia have been cleansed and assessed, the child should be asked to void and kept in the emergency department until she is able to do so. An inability to void or gross hematuria is indication for further assessment. If there is any question of disruption of the urethra, a catheter should not be passed, to avoid exacerbating the injury, and immediate urologic consultation should be requested.

If there is any reason to suspect sexual abuse, the child protection authorities must be notified, and the examination should include the collection of medicolegal evidence. Collection of evidence is not, in itself, adequate justification to subject a child to the further risk of general anesthesia. Although ideally this examination is done by a member of a skilled child abuse team, sometimes it may fall to a less experienced person. Regardless of who examines the child, a principle must be to assist the child and not contribute to the insult.

Vaginal Bleeding

Vaginal bleeding is a common complaint in childhood and one that causes a great deal of concern. These children usually require referral to a gynecologist for a definitive diagnosis, but examination in the emergency department may disclose the cause.

Vaginal bleeding in the newborn is most often physiologic, as a result of maternal estrogen withdrawal. If estrogen withdrawal is the working diagnosis, there should be evidence of hormonal effect such as breast tissue and pale engorged vaginal mucosa. Bleeding disorders are uncommon in this age group but should be considered. Vitamin K is routinely given to the newborn, but it is worth ensuring that the parents did not refuse the treatment.

Precocious puberty may occur with vaginal bleeding, although most commonly other evidence of maturation will have preceded the bleeding and will be evident on examination. At the very least, a pale estrogenized vaginal mucosa will be seen, and cytology from the vagina will confirm the hormonal effect. Referral should be made to look for the source of estrogen. Central precocious puberty may be idiopathic but may well be pathologic. Exogenous hormone should be considered since children have been known to eat birth control pills. Ovarian tumors may be estrogen producing and should be ruled out.

Urethral prolapse is not uncommon in young girls aged 4 to 6. The bright red tender mass may be mistaken for a traumatized hymen or for a tumor. Many will respond to sitz baths and topical estrogen, but others will persist and require surgical management.

Condyloma acuminata are an increasingly commonly described cause of vaginal bleeding. In infancy, condyloma acuminata have a lush, proliferative appearance in contrast to the dry, wartlike lesions found in older patients. These may be transmitted perinatally, particularly in infants, but sexual abuse must be considered.

Vulvovaginitis is common but is a diagnosis of exclusion. When bleeding is present, referral is warranted to assess the vagina and rule out foreign body or vaginal tumor. Poor hygiene, the susceptibility of the unestrogenized mucosa to infection and minor irritation, and the activities of childhood all play a part in the frequency of this complaint, and if more serious pathology has been excluded, conservative management can be recommended. Agents that lead to excessive drying of the skin, such as lengthy soaks or baking soda baths, should be avoided. Scrupulous skin care and hydration using agents such as colloidal oatmeal will be more successful.

Vulvar skin conditions may be missed in childhood, and it is important to look for eczema, psoriasis, lichen planus, and lichen sclerosus et atrophicus, all of which can affect genital skin in childhood.

Vaginal tumors are the most serious possibility to be considered; sarcoma botryoides classically occurs with vaginal bleeding and has an appearance of grapelike vesicles. Fortunately this is a rare tumor.

Trauma or child abuse must always be considered. Careful history taking and visual inspection are critical to making the diagnosis. Suspicion of abuse mandates notification of child welfare authorities.

Dysfunctional Uterine Bleeding

Menstrual disorders are common in adolescence, and excessive bleeding is a common presentation in emergency departments. A systematic approach should be adopted in assessing these patients and should follow from an understanding of adolescent menstrual physiology.

Menarche, the first menstrual flow, is almost always the shedding of an endometrium stimulated by rising levels of estrogen throughout puberty, without ovulation. At first, many cycles may likewise be anovulatory. Until the feedback pathways are well established, teenagers are likely to fail to ovulate from time to time and may return to an irregular pattern even after many apparently regular menses.

Other causes of excessive, irregular, or acyclic bleeding that must always be considered are bleeding disorders, pregnancy, and infection. Metabolic and neoplastic conditions may also occur with dysfunctional bleeding.

The initial history should include age of menarche and a detailed history of the menstrual pattern to date, episodes of faintness or syncope, history of bleeding or bruising, sexual history, and functional inquiry, including weight loss or gain, energy and activity level, and sleep disturbance.

Investigation

The primary laboratory investigation is a complete blood count. A hemoglobin level is not sufficient because both the white cell and the platelet counts are needed to rule out blood dyscrasias. Prothrombin time, partial thromboplastin time, and bleeding times are reasonable tests for any patient whose complaint is sufficiently severe as to bring her to the emergency department.

Bleeding may occur in any early pregnancy but is a warning sign for either ectopic pregnancy or spontaneous abortion. A sensitive urinary pregnancy test or screening serum beta human chorionic gonadotropin should be routinely ordered.

Cervicitis or pelvic inflammatory disease may produce irregular bleeding. In a sexually active patient, or in any patient in whom pelvic pain, fever, or leukocytosis is present, cultures for bacteria and

Chlamydia should be obtained. Enzyme-linked immunosorbent assay screening tests for *Chlamydia* are a popular alternative to culture techniques but may not be as reliable in the presence of vaginal bleeding. The laboratory will provide information on the test that is being used locally.

Acyclic bleeding can also indicate an underlying malignant process. Leukemia and idiopathic thrombocytopenic purpura may produce dysfunctional bleeding, and cervical or endometrial cancer may occur in young age groups. A prolonged history of menstrual irregularity, intermenstrual bleeding, or early age of first sexual exposure are risk factors which should lead to a gynecologic consultation.

Metabolic causes of dysfunctional bleeding that may be encountered in adolescence include diabetes mellitus, hyperthyroidism, and hypothyroidism. The systems review should help, but a urine dipstick for glucose and screening thyroid function studies are reasonable in an adolescent with a history of dysfunctional bleeding. Prolactinemia may be associated with oligomenorrhea or amenorrhea but is unlikely to appear in the emergency department. Cushing's syndrome is uncommon but should be borne in mind.

Management

Prolonged Bleeding

The typical presentation of prolonged bleeding is for a young teenager to come in with a history of bleeding of several weeks' duration that is at times heavy and at other times just spotting but that never goes away. Her cycle up to that time may or may not have been regular. Because of the indolent course, she is usually hemodynamically stable, although she may be quite anemic. In a reliable patient if investigation fails to reveal any other organic cause, outpatient management may be recommended using monophasic combination oral contraceptives, such as Min-Ovral, Ovral, or Ortho 1/35 tablets, assuming there is no contraindication to their use. These should be provided with instructions to take two every 6 hours until bleeding is controlled then to take one tablet daily until the packet is finished. Antinauseants may be needed, either in suppository or transdermal form. The patient should be warned to expect a heavy flow at the end of one pack and directed to start a new package, one pill daily, 1 week later. A follow-up appointment should be made in 2 to 3 weeks for continuing supervision.

Heavy Flow

The presentation of heavy flow bleeding is more dramatic, with the onset of heavy flow with the passage of clots per vagina, and is frequently accompanied by syncope or faintness. In these cases, it is particularly important to exclude bleeding disorders and complications of pregnancy. Some may be managed as outpatients. However, if there are any signs of hemodynamic instability, if hemoglobin level is less than 90 g per liter, or if the patient is saturating a pad in less than an hour, admission to control the blood loss is indicated. Management includes fluid replacement and hormonal control of bleeding, either with combination contraceptive tablets, two every 4 hours or with intravenous Premarin, 25 mg every 4 hours. Bleeding should be controlled within 24 to 36 hours. If bleeding persists, an examination under anesthesia and dilation and curettage may be necessary to rule out organic pathology.

Sexually Transmitted Disease

The diagnosis and treatment of sexually transmitted disease (STD) in the adolescent age group is not dealt with in any detail in this chapter because it can be found in any manual of adult gynecologic emergency care. However, some important points that bear emphasis when assessing teenagers are mentioned.

Teenaged women are at great risk for sexually transmitted infection not only because of the risk taking, but also their poorly developed judgment of others so characteristic of this age group. They are much less likely to have been using contraceptives or barriers in a consistent fashion and less likely to be in a stable relationship. Cultures to rule out STDs should be obtained routinely. There is a high incidence of multiple sexually transmitted infections coexisting. *Chlamydia* is more difficult to culture than is *Neisseria gonorrhea* and should be assumed to be present if gonorrhea is diagnosed. Reporting guidelines to public health authorities may vary according to jurisdiction, but most STDs do require reporting and contact tracing.

Because of poor compliance with medications, gonococcal cervicitis or asymptomatic infection should be treated with single-dose therapy followed by treatment for *Chlamydia*. There is no place for outpatient management of pelvic inflammatory disease. Any patient with suspected pelvic inflammatory disease should be admitted for definitive diagnosis and intravenous antibiotic therapy.

The presence of a sexually transmitted infection in a child requires immediate reporting to child welfare authorities. When parents are told that their child has a sexually transmitted disease, they are often very concerned about the consequences to the child's potential fertility. However, because of the unestrogenized state of the genital tract, young children seem to be spared the risk of pelvic inflammatory disease and the complications that go with it. As a consequence, the psychological trauma generally leaves far more scars than the infection, once treated.

Imperforate Hymen with Hematocolpos

Rarely the hymen remains intact until menarche when the child may present with abdominal pain, lower abdominal mass, and a bluish bulge filling the vaginal introitus. Direct referral to gynecology permits operative excision of the membrane and careful exploration of the vagina to rule out a second septum higher up. The intact hymen should never be needled.

The Extremities

The Hip

Examination of the Hip

In the emergency department, a practical "mini-examination" of the hip, including the main points but omitting many of the specialized components of a complete detailed orthopaedic assessment, can be a very useful tool. When they are recorded on the chart, the findings of such a mini-examination indicate to anyone reviewing the chart that the examining physician knew something about examining hips. Too often the hip is examined with the same approach and with the same recorded terms that are used in evaluating knees, elbows, or finger joints.

The examination described here is based on an understanding of the abductor mechanism of the hip and a knowledge of the anatomy of the hip joint capsule. For practical purposes, this examination applies to inflammatory disease into which category fit the bulk of hip lesions that we currently see. We rarely now see children with abductor paralysis, such as those who had poliomyelitis years before, or children who are walking on untreated congenitally dislocated hips. On the other hand, the slipped femoral capital epiphysis must be thought of separately. Legg-Calvé-Perthes disease should be included also, but when a child with this disease presents in the emergency department, he or she usually has inflammation.

Abductor Mechanism

When it contracts, the gluteus medius abducts the hip by pulling closer together the iliac crest and the greater trochanter. This action swings the leg out laterally when the subject stands on the opposite leg or holds the pelvis level when the subject stands on the leg in question while holding the other foot off the floor.

The Trendelenburg sign is the visible dropping of the opposite side of the pelvis when the subject attempts to stand solely on the affected leg. This sign was frequently seen when many late cases of poliomyelitis or untreated congenital hip dislocation were still being encountered. It is now rarely seen in the emergency department of a pediatric hospital, where currently most hip disease is inflammatory. In the presence of a painful inflamed hip, one is unable to persuade a child to stand with all weight on the painful leg. On the other hand, children with sore hips do display the gait reminiscent of the polio victim. This is commonly called the Trendelenburg gait, although Trendelenburg himself never described the gait.

The Trendelenburg gait is characterized by a shift of the upper body toward the side of the inflamed hip when weight is borne solely on that leg. This body shift decreases the weight borne by that hip. In other words, the patient "takes weight off the sore hip by leaning over it." This apparent paradox is explained by picturing the pelvis as a lever with the body weight pressing down on one end and the gluteus medius pulling down on the other end. The hip joint itself is the fulcrum and carries the total downward weight sustained by both segments of the pelvic lever. Hence, the weight borne by the hip with every step is the arithmetic sum of the two forces acting on the pelvis, which amounts to twice or more the body weight.

For this reason, a subject bearing weight, however briefly, on an inflamed hip will lean the body toward that side, bringing the center of gravity over the fulcrum. This removes the need for the abductor to contract to keep the individual upright. The result of the body shift is to bring the total weight borne by the sore hip down to an amount equal to that supported by the sacrum. This is one-half or less than one-half of the weight borne by that hip during normal walking.

Although the body shift displayed by a child with mild synovitis is frequently very slight, it is usually easily displayed when sought and remains a very important clue to help one identify the hip as the source of a child's symptoms.

Hip Joint Capsule

Why does a child hold the hip in flexion and external rotation when the joint is full of fluid under pressure, as in acute synovitis or septic arthritis? The reason for this is that this posture gives maximum volume in the joint and hence minimum pressure and discomfort. In the anatomic position, the capsular fibers spiral downward and inward so that externally rotating the leg unwinds them, increasing the capacity.

How has this normal but unexpected configuration evolved? It is known that in the developing embryo all four limb buds appear initially with the palmar or plantar surfaces directly anteriorly. The palmar surface of the arms remains directed forward, whereas the legs soon demonstrate an internal rotation of 180 degrees, which turns the plantar surfaces to face posteriorly. This embryonic transition represents the phylogenetic or evolutionary change that occurred as humans' arboreal ancestors became terrestrial quadrupeds, with soles of the feet now contacting the ground.

The result of this capsular configuration is that the hip is nearly at its limit of internal rotation in the "normal" anatomic position, and even a small amount of joint fluid renders further internal rotation painful. Loss of internal rotation is a sensitive and delicate indicator of fluid in the joint and is sometimes the last indication of inflammation persisting after all other signs have resolved during the recovery phase.

A further evolutionary process that ensured was gradual extension of the hips, enabling what were hitherto terrestrial quadripeds to become upright bipeds. Extension, however, has resulted in a hip joint the anterior capsule of which is short, tough, and thick, markedly limiting further extension, and the posterior capsule of which is long and redundant, permitting a great deal of flexion. With even a small effusion, the lack of redundancy anteriorly of necessity results in a degree of flexion. This produces the clinical observation of limitation of extension, or what is commonly called a flexion deformity or flexion contracture.

How does a small child with a slight flexion deformity due to a small effusion still manage to stand upright with legs straight and feet flat on the floor? The child does it by rotating the pelvis forward, thus permitting flexion of both hips, while at the same time hyperextending the lumbar spine, which enables the trunk to remain in the upright position. The lumbar lordosis so caused masks the hip flexion. Consequently, the clinician should watch for excessive lumbar lordosis because it may indicate a hip flexion deformity. When the child is supine, lumbar lordosis can again hide the hip flexion, particularly if the buttocks have sunk into a soft mattress, obscuring the space under the lumbar spine. To demonstrate this, one must remove the lumbar hyperextension that has been masking the hip flexion deformity. It is an easy matter to bring the good leg up over the patient's body, flexing it at hip and knee, until the examiner's hand, placed behind the lumbar spine, is squeezed between bed and back. When the compensatory lordosis has been completely obliterated in this way, the painful hip will automatically flex to a degree which corresponds to the hip flexion deformity. This is Thomas' test. When Thomas' test is positive, one can conclude that there is limitation of extension, or hip flexion deformity.

Three Signs

Three signs—Trendelenburg gait, limitation of internal rotation, and Thomas' test—form a practical examination routine and should be on the chart as a bare minimum for any patient suspected to have hip disease, unless, for some reason, there is contraindication to attempt any one of them. For example, one should not have a child up walking if one suspects a partially slipped femoral capital epiphysis. It is also very unlikely that a child with septic arthritis would be willing or able to walk.

It should be emphasized that the child with an early slip of the femoral capital epiphysis will quite possibly not demonstrate any of the three signs described. Unless there is excessive joint fluid, internal rotation should not be limited. The epiphysis shifts posteriorly when it slips, so extension will be increased if anything, and certainly not decreased. Unless pain is significant at the time, any limp may be virtually undetectable. For this reason, any child between 9 and 16 years of age who has a history of pain that may have its origin in the hip (i.e., located in any or all of hip, thigh, or knee) or who has an unexplained limp, even in the absence of any detectable signs pointing to hip pathology, should be assumed to have an early slip of a femoral epiphysis, which, if allowed to slip further, could result in disastrous long-term consequences. In such a child, appropriate radiographs must be obtained and carefully reviewed before weight-bearing is permitted. Even very slight slippage, often recognized only on the lateral (frog) view, requires urgent orthopaedic treatment.

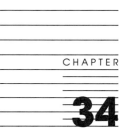

34

Inflammation of the Hip

Monarticular Synovitis (Transient Synovitis)

Monarticular synovitis is a nonbacterial inflammation of the joint, the cause of which is largely unknown, although some have suggested a viral etiology for at least some examples. It occurs in children between 3 and 10 years of age and is much more common in boys than in girls. The inflammation results in fluid accumulation within the synovial space, pain and restriction of movement, and a degree of systemic reaction, which, however, is usually very slight if detectable at all.

The history is usually that of pain with activity that increases over a day or so until it may be so severe as to prevent walking. Although the pain is usually in the groin, it may be located in the thigh or knee or any combination thereof. There may be slight fever.

Inspection will usually reveal a Trendelenburg gait, although the shift of the upper body over the affected hip may be very slight. Some children demonstrate what seems to be a combination of antalgic and Trendelenburg gaits.

When supine, the child will lie with hip flexed, externally rotated, and abducted. Although the flexion may not be obvious, excessive lordosis and a positive Thomas' test will demonstrate that there is a flexion deformity. Usually internal rotation is particularly limited, as are all other movements but to a lesser degree. Occasionally, in the child with very mild synovitis who manifests few abnormal physical findings, slight limitation of internal rotation may be the only detectable sign to indicate the joint effusion. Even in instances of severe inflammation, it is usually possible to put the hip quite vigorously through the mid-range of flexion-extension with very little discomfort.

In synovitis, evidence of joint effusion can sometimes be noted on radiograph. However, the observations are usually equivocal, and it is certainly permissible to omit radiography in mild cases, provided that the decision is made to obtain radiographs if signs of inflammation do not subside rapidly. However, because many cases of Legg-Calvé-Perthes disease have a clinical presentation with all the characteristics of synovitis, some recommend routine radiographic assessment of the hips to rule out this disease. A child who has moderate or severe synovitis should undergo radiographic examination, as should the child with a second attack of synovitis, however mild it might be, if he or she did not undergo radiographic examination initially. The radiographic manifestations of Legg-Calvé-Perthes disease may be delayed for many months, so in that rare instance when there is urgency in establishing that a child with normal x-ray films does not have Legg-Calvé-Perthes disease, which might subsequently become manifest, a bone scan is worthwhile.

The chief diagnostic concern is the need to be confident the child does not have early septic arthritis. Provided that the child has not received antibiotics before referral, the course of septic arthritis is generally one of rapid worsening. Conversely, the rapidly improving picture of most children with synovitis who are put to bed is an important argument against septic arthritis. Furthermore, in bacterial arthritis, physical examination of the hip reveals severe pain with any movement. The ability to move the hip through the mid-range of flexion-extension in even quite severe synovitis provides useful information in helping to rule out sepsis.

Although systemic manifestations are usually absent in toxic synovitis, slight fever is compatible with the diagnosis, and there may even be a slight granulocytic leukocytosis, although if elevation in temperature or white cells count is marked, septic arthritis, must be carefully considered. A very elevated sedimentation rate, i.e., over 60, is frequently seen in hip joint sepsis.

Differentiation between monarticular synovitis and septic arthritis hinges clinically on the intensity of the inflammatory reaction, both local and systemic. This judgment is based largely on one's experience, can be very difficult to make, and has potentially disastrous consequences if incorrect. For this reason, there must never be hesitation to refer to an orthopaedic consultant should there be any doubt. Joint aspiration and examination of such fluid as is obtained provide the definitive diagnosis. This is ideally carried out under general anesthesia, thus permitting immediate joint exploration and drainage if purulent fluid is obtained.

Rheumatoid arthritis rarely begins in the hip, but when it does, it may closely simulate toxic synovitis. On the other hand, one does not expect rheumatoid arthritis to show the rapid improvement within the first 24 hours of treatment that synovitis normally displays. Nevertheless, should improvement be slow or if other joints become involved, laboratory investigation looking for collagen-vascular disease will be required.

The treatment of most children with synovitis consists of bed rest to minimize weight bearing until symptoms have largely resolved. Rapid improvement can be anticipated, and almost complete recovery rarely requires more than a week. If there is not steady improvement over the first day or so, reassessment of the diagnosis is warranted. Patients with mild cases can be treated at home. Patients with more severe disease should probably be admitted to the hospital to permit careful observation lest the diagnosis need be revised.

The use of salicylates or other anti-inflammatory drugs is questionable. The normally rapid improvement in symptoms and signs of monarticular synovitis does not generally justify specific therapy. Observed improvement in the clinical picture is important in substantiating the diagnosis, and one might well not know whether to attribute improvement while on such a pharmaceutical agent to the medication or to the expected course of disease. Observation without medication is recommended.

Recurrent attacks of synovitis are seen from time to time, although this situation should alert one to the possibility of Legg-Calvé-Perthes disease.

Septic Arthritis of the Hip

Infections of bone or joint are very serious and have the potential for permanent crippling. In the preantibiotic era, up to 25 percent of patients died of the associated septicemia and metastatic abscesses. Hence, with our advanced knowledge of the disease and current availability of effective antibiotic therapy, all efforts must be directed toward early diagnosis of such infections to permit current therapy to exert its maximum effect. In spite of excellent therapeutic tools, long-term complications are encountered all too frequently as a result of late diagnosis and delayed institution of treatment or inadequate utilization of the methods and drugs available.

Bacterial infection of a joint is usually due to septic extension from an area of staphylococcal osteomyelitis in the end of one of the articulating long bones. Hematogenous osteomyelitis of any long bone generally begins in the metaphysis near the epiphyseal plate. Here local bone infection spreads in several directions, one of which is toward and through the cortex. When the metaphysis is completely intracapsular, as is the case with the hip, infection progressing beyond the cortex immediately involves the joint space. Where the physis and metaphysis of the bone are extracapsular the joints are not immediately involved by extraosseous extension of infection from the bone. Consequently, such joints are much less often the site of septic arthritis than are those joints in which the physis and metaphysis are intracapsular, such as the hip or elbow.

As is the case with hematogenous osteomyelitis, the most common organism in the septic hip is the *Staphylococcus aureus*. Other less common organisms recovered are *Streptococcus hemolyticus*, *Streptococcus pneumoniae*, *Haemophilus influenzae*, *Salmonella*, *Neisseria gonorrhoeae*, and *Brucella*. However, these probably cause no more than 10 percent of all septic arthritides and are thought to do so by way of the direct hematogenous route, not via the intermediate stage of osteomyelitis of the adjacent bone.

The course of established staphylococcal sepsis in the hip joint is one of rapid progression. Pus within the capsule soon causes destruction of the articular cartilage through the effect of enzyme products, the acidic pH of the pus, and pressure. Unfortunately articular cartilage does not regenerate, and the degree of destruction produced by the infection is permanent.

The septic effusion under pressure also causes edema and weakening of the capsular fibers. Particularly in infancy this increased capsular laxity may result in dislocation. Furthermore, the pressure itself may occlude the retinacular blood vessels and those traveling in the round ligament, in turn resulting in ischemic necrosis of the femoral head. In the infant with a septic hip, total loss of the femoral head is a well-recognized outcome.

All these disastrous results of septic arthritis of the hip may be prevented or at least minimized by early recognition and prompt institution of the appropriate treatment.

The diagnosis of septic arthritis of the hip in infancy can be difficult. However, any sick baby in whom the diagnosis is in question must be assessed for the possibility of an infection of bone or joint in the same way that meningitis is always looked for.

Inspection will reveal that one extremity is not being used as much as the others or not at all. When that extremity is a leg, the diagnosis of a septic hip must be at the top of the list. The hip will be held in external rotation and flexion, and there will be evidence of marked pain on any movement of the joint. If there are any radiographic findings, one can assume that the disease is well advanced and will have severe permanent effects. Radiographic changes in bone begin to appear after a week at the earliest, and completely successful treatment is possible only if it is started well before that time.

Systemic signs are minimal until the local disease has progressed. Although fever and leukocytosis can be expected, these may be slight or even nonexistent in the young infant.

In the older child, early diagnosis is usually much easier to reach with accuracy. Constant pain in the hip, with extreme pain on any movement, in a child who is likely to be febrile and who demonstrates some degree of systemic toxicity should lead to the presumption of septic arthritis. Once more, radiographic changes such as localized bony destruction and periosteal new bone do not show up for a week or more and are indication of an advanced stage of the disease and a less than optimum outcome.

Unfortunately inadequate dosage of antibiotics for a presumed mild infection of some sort can mask the developing signs of septic arthritis by suppressing the disease without killing the organisms. For this reason, the clinician must be alert to the possibility of a serious infection, such as an infected hip, in the child who has been receiving antibiotics for a "cold" but who also displays a clinical picture, however mild, which might be produced by a low-grade smoldering septic joint.

In such situations, aggressive therapy, both medical and surgical, is required to minimize the risk of permanent sequelae.

Because purulent arthritis requires prompt orthopaedic intervention, immediate referral is necessary whenever a septic hip is a reasonable possibility.

Diagnostic confirmation by joint aspiration and examination of the fluid obtained is the first step in definitive treatment. This is ideally performed under general anesthesia and image intensification fluoroscopy by the same surgeon who, if pus is obtained, can immediately move the child into the open operating theater for arthrotomy and drainage. If the attempted aspiration fails, surgical exploration is also required. Only if water-clear fluid is obtained can joint sepsis be eliminated.

Immediately after several samples for culture have been obtained, high dosage of the appropriate antibiotic, preferably given by vein, is essential. This, more than anything else, has been responsible for controlling the morbidity and mortality from septicemia. On the other hand, antibiotic therapy is adjunctive treatment only for the hip disease itself and must never be used as an excuse for delay in surgical drainage, for which septic arthritis is an absolute indication.

If immediate transfer to orthopaedic care is not possible, the primary physician is advised to base continuing treatment on telephone advice from an orthopaedic consultant.

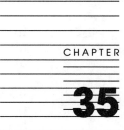

35

Limp and Leg Pain

Limp

Abnormalities of gait possess many different forms and arise from many different causes. Most would be included in the following broad groups:

1. *Neurologic*—muscle weakness, hypotonic or spastic; incoordination (cerebellar); sensory loss
2. *Mechanical*—limb deformity, leg length discrepancy, joint abnormality, restriction of movement
3. *Psychological*—hysteria, mimicry
4. *Pain-induced*—pain arising in the involved extremity: either from causes in the hip or produced in sites below the hip; pain from disease elsewhere: spinal, abdominal

With few exceptions, any limp displayed in the emergency department by a child who normally has no limp is the result of pain, and it is the job of the emergency physician to find the site and nature of the painful lesion.

Because acute spinal disease is unusual in children, gait disturbance due to acute spinal conditions is rare. However, spinal osteomyelitis, disk disease, contusion of paraspinal musculature, or compression fracture may result in a careful, rigid, guarded gait that is exaggerated on the side of the discomfort. In these cases, examination will usually reveal flattening of the lumbar spine, increased paraspinal tone, and spinal movements that are limited by pain. That the spine is the source of the discomfort should also be easily identified from the history of the symptoms.

Intra-abdominal inflammation, e.g., acute appendicitis, should be considered if the child walks with a visibly flexed hip, steps very gingerly on the affected side, and holds the abdomen with the hand. The history of abdominal pain and vomiting, with signs of peritoneal irritation on examination, should identify the intra-abdominal location of the lesion.

The vast majority of children who walk with an acute limp do so because of a "sore leg." The gait produced is of two general types, depending on whether the hip is sore or part of the leg below the hip is sore.

The limp commonly called an "antalgic gait" is adopted in response to discomfort arising anywhere in the leg below the hip. Although the most frequent causes are injuries to the foot or ankle, foreign bodies in the sole of the foot; "toddlers' tibial fractures"; and any painful conditions involving the thigh, knee, or lower leg are possibilities. The antalgic gait is the result of a desire to bear as little weight for as short a time as possible on the offending member. Hence, the weight-bearing phase is shortened, and weight is returned to the other foot as soon as possible. The sore extremity is permitted to bear weight for only as long as it takes to get the other foot back up under the individual again.

Following a traumatic episode, an antalgic limp implies pain arising in some part of the leg. Efforts must be made to identify the site of tenderness so that radiographs can be restricted to the part involved. Although it may be difficult to decide what part of the leg is sore in an inconsolably crying child, one can usually do so. The importance of doing this and the methods of accomplishing it are discussed in Chapter 40.

On the other hand, a sore hip will almost always result in what is commonly called a Trendelenburg gait. The subject who has a painful hip shifts the upper body over the sore hip whenever he or she bears weight on that side. The subject leans over the sore hip to remove weight from the hip. In essence, the hip is carrying least weight when the center of gravity of the subject's body is situated directly over it. Further discussion of this can be found in Chapter 33.

The child with mild monarticular synovitis may shift the upper body to a very slight degree, whereas the adult with severe osteoarthritis of the hip will usually lean markedly over the affected hip with each step. When the hip pain is severe, the subject may not only lean over the hip when bearing weight on it, but also may shorten the weight-bearing phase of the gait. This could be described as a combination of hip limp and antalgic limp.

Leg Pain

From time to time a child is seen who has persistent mild leg pain or limp following trauma but who has no other detectable physical findings. This will usually be a young child who has a slight limp following seemingly minor trauma. In these cases, it is reasonable to temporize for a few days before any investigation is undertaken. However, if there is not steady improvement, radiographs are warranted.

Occasionally a bone tumor can cause persisting pain in an extremity, and for this reason unexplained extremity pain which persists does require investigation at some stage. Avoiding unnecessary radiographs is desirable, and no harm will come from delaying the diagnosis of a bone tumor for 3 or 4 days while waiting to see if the pain lessens. However, one must not lose track of this sort of patient because the situation must be resolved before closing the case. Characteristically pain from a malignant bone tumor is constant, progressively more severe, and present when not bearing weight.

Growing Pains

Occasionally the 3- to 5-year old will be seen who regularly awakens at night with pains in the legs, usually of a crampy nature and situated in the calf muscles. When seen the following day, the child seems perfectly normal after careful examination. For want of any better label, this syndrome has often been called "growing pains"; the name is perhaps more related to old superstitions than to extremity growth. On the other hand, appositional bone growth occurs partially through internal remodeling, the mechanism for which may be largely through microfracturing. Growing pains may reflect the effect of intense activity superimposed on the remodeling process and so may be indirectly related to growth.

This complaint is sufficiently common and so characteristic that reassurance alone is justified, unless the pains persist for weeks. This type of discomfort is not suggestive of bone tumor and does not warrant extensive investigation, unless one is pushed into it by the duration of the discomfort.

36

Infections

Infections Around Fingernails or Toenails

Recurrent Infected Ingrown Toenails: Acute Attack

The classic example of a periungual infection is the so-called infected ingrown toenail, which is a common nuisance condition for which the pathogenesis is poorly understood and for which there is much disagreement as to appropriate treatment. The lack of solid scientific knowledge regarding this condition is evident when one is exposed to the countless remedies, lay and otherwise, that are advocated for this condition. The emphasis in this chapter is on one underlying principal pathogenesis, and except for instances in which the nail requires surgical removal, it embodies one specific treatment procedure on the basis of that pathogenesis.

With only a few exceptions, superficial inflammatory lesions on the body surface heal spontaneously. However, one of those exceptions, perhaps the most common, is inflammation in the presence of an associated foreign body. One cannot expect the small laceration on the back of the hand to heal if there is a piece of wood embedded in it. Herein lies the fundamental pathology of the ingrown toenail. Because the nail itself is dead tissue, it behaves as a foreign body and has the same effect on tissue inflammation as does a wooden splinter, a retained sponge after laparotomy, or a bony sequestrum. Not only is the foreign body the reason for the perpetuation of the local inflammation, but also treatment hinges on the recognition that this condition is a foreign body disease. Separation of the foreign body and the inflamed tissues, one from the other, is the basis for successful therapy.

Many different situations may precipitate the initial lesion. A blow to the toe can cause a scratch or tiny laceration along the margin of the nail, or a superficial tear beside the nail can be the result of efforts to remove a hangnail. Alternatively the patient may have produced a small traumatic lesion when picking the toenail. Lateral compression from tight shoes may have compressed the soft tissue against the nail edge to the extent that a shallow erosion has been created.

Once there is an epithelial defect, the healing process is immediately compromised by the presence of the foreign body. Persistent subacute inflammation is the usual outcome, with granulation tissue being an important feature of it. Superimposed infection is inevitable, and both purulent drainage and cellulitis in the adjacent toe tissue can be expected.

The term "ingrown nail" is a misnomer. The nail does not grow laterally because there is no germinal matrix extending out the middle of the nail to generate growth laterally. The germinal matrix from which the nail grows lies across the proximal end of the nail and produces distally directed growth only. The appearance of ingrowing results from the edema of the tissue lateral to the nail, causing it to heap up over the edge of the nail.

The clinical picture of an early ingrown toenail is readily recognized by those patients who have had many attacks previously and seek to learn how to prevent recurrences. Tenderness of the tissues lateral to the nail, very slight at first but progressing, with associated redness and edema, heralds the onset of full-blown foreign body inflammation, usually at the site of some minor traumatic lesion of which the patient may have been unaware. Granulations appear as the process advances and have the appearance of small pieces of liver protruding beside the nail. Infection becomes superimposed so that the drainage becomes purulent and adjacent cellulitis develops.

Although surgical removal of part or all of the nail is necessary when treating advanced cases, management of early cases consists of removing the inflamed tissues from the foreign body. Nontoothed thumb forceps, an orange stick, a tongue blade split to produce a picklike end, and even a toothpick whittled to produce a flat surface can all be used to push the inflamed tissues away from the nail. This develops a crevice along the edge of the nail. In the very early cases, repeating this procedure several times a day, after a shower or a bath, will usually result in rapid and complete resolution of the inflammation. However, usually more intervention is needed. After each manipulation is carried out, a strip of cotton batten twisted into a wormlike form is packed into the crevice beside the nail by means of the tool used to retract the tissues. Several times each day, again preferably after a shower or bath, the pack is removed and replaced with clean packing. The pack can be held in place by a loosely applied bandage.

One will be surprised how easy it is to displace the inflamed tissues laterally and establish the crevice or crack into which the packing is placed. Furthermore, after the physician has carried out the procedure for the first time, it becomes much easier and less painful to move the inflamed tissues and hence much easier for the child or a parent to carry on at home. Teenagers usually manage to do this very well when they are reminded that the assiduousness of their manipulations may well be instrumental in removing the need for surgical excision of the nail.

This procedure will normally result in subsidence of the inflammation within a few days. If no improvement is noted, one is still able to proceed to surgical removal of a strip of nail. However, the patient will have learned the appropriate treatment to use after the nail has regenerated and when the next attack is just starting. The procedure of holding the tissues away from the foreign body works best in the very early stages and has its greatest advantage in preventing further progression of the inflammation when early redness and tenderness are first noted.

For many surgeons, the treatment for adults who have had recurrent attacks of infected ingrown toenails is removal of a strip of nail and excision of the underlying germinal matrix to prevent regrowth of that portion of the nail. These same surgeons will often tend to proceed in like fashion when treating the teenager who has had only one or two attacks. It must be emphasized that there is no indication for matrix ablation in the child. To narrow the nail permanently in a child who has merely had several attacks of infected ingrown toenail is excessive and unnecessary and is usually indication that neither surgeon nor patient has tried rigorously enough to prevent early inflammations from progressing to the stage requiring nail excision.

Recurrent attacks of infected ingrown toenails are common. Even when such a patient has had the toenail surgically removed, further attacks can occur once the nail has grown back in. For this reason, there are major benefits in having a patient learn the manipulations necessary to separate the tissues from the foreign body. This provides the patient with the tool to prevent subsequent attacks from progressing beyond the very early stages.

Acute Paronychia

Infections around the margins of the nail are common, basically because normal tissues do not deal effectively with small traumatic lesions or localized infections when abutting closely up against the nail, which behaves as a foreign body. Infections elsewhere usually progress spontaneously to drainage and resolution. This does not happen along the nail edge, and surgical drainage is necessary much more often.

Acute paronychia, or "runaround," appears as an area of acute inflammation in a portion of the soft tissue immediately adjacent to the nail. As paronychia progresses, it may even extend around much of the nail. In the very early stages, gentle retraction of the cuticle with thumb forceps or part of a tongue depressor may achieve adequate drainage, without the need for any anesthesia.

With many moderately early cases of paronychia, drainage under digital block anesthesia is satisfactory, although injections into the finger should be avoided when the infection is particularly acute because one should not be injecting into the area of the neurovascular bundles when it can be predicted that the lymphatics will be loaded with staphylococci. Brachial plexus block, venous block, and general anesthesia are all options.

The eponychia is elevated with a scalpel blade or fine pointed scissors in the area of the inflammation, thus releasing any pus situated beneath the tissue. Care should be taken merely to elevate the eponychia and not to incise more deeply, unless there is indication of pus within the tissues. Removal of the nail is necessary in some cases but certainly not in all, particularly if there is no indication of pus beneath the nail edge. Often this cannot be determined until the finger is anesthetized and the abscess space has been entered.

In advanced cases of paronychia, in which pus appears around most of the nail and there is pus below parts of the nail, adequate drainage necessitates removal of the nail as well.

Antibiotics are useful in finger infections such as acute paronychia as adjuncts only. An appropriate antistaphylococcal agent may decrease the risk of serious complications, such as lymphangitis, adenitis, or septicemia, and it will be effective in dealing with associated cellulitis. However, paronychia requires surgical treatment, and the decision to drain must be made first and independent of any decision regarding antibacterial therapy. Although many clinicians will begin the medication several hours before the surgical procedure is carried out to achieve an effective blood level prior to surgery, one should not use antibiotic therapy in the hope of avoiding drainage.

Chronic Paronychia

In cases of chronic paronychia, one will occasionally encounter a baby who has had persistent redness and crusting around a fingernail for some weeks. There will usually be little or no pain associated with it and little drainage. Little is known about the reason for the development of such low-grade inflammations which are recalcitrant to treatment, although it has been suggested that many of these are at least in part due to the tissue maceration resulting from persistent thumb or finger sucking. That this condition is not often seen after the age of 2 years supports this hypothesis.

Although the redness of the involved tissue can be quite striking, the tenderness is usually minimal. This permits easy removal of the crusting and fibrinous exudate with thumb forceps. Manual retraction of the periungual soft tissues, as is done in ingrown toenails, exposes the tissues to the air, lets them dry, and removes any damaging effect of the nail itself.

If thumb or finger sucking can than be kept to a minimum, improvement can be expected. Complete resolution may take a number of weeks.

Subungual Abscess

Pus under a fingernail or toenail can result from extension of paronychia or infection in a subungual collection of blood. It may even develop after a subungual hematoma has been drained (possibly drained inadequately). At any rate, subungual pus is indication for nail removal under the appropriate form of anesthesia. When the nail has been removed, rapid clearing of infection can be expected, with or without adjunctive antibiotic therapy. Rarely the collection of pus may be so localized and so close to the distal edge of the nail that merely cutting a V from the edge can expose the abscess to permit adequate drainage.

Parents are always concerned that trauma, infection, and drainage procedures may result in subsequent abnormal nail regrowth. Fortunately most traumatic insults, most hematomas, and most collections of pus are located under the middle or distal portion of the nail and because the germinal matrix is situated proximally, it is usually uninvolved. Even when a laceration crosses the matrix proximally, the late outcome is usually satisfactory, provided that the deformity in the nail bed is kept to a minimum.

Specific Infections of the Extremities

Pulp Space Infection

Often called a "felon" or a "whitlow," a pulp space infection occurs in the touch pad of the terminal digit of a finger, where fibrous septa between the terminal phalanx and the skin produce tiny compartments within which pressure can build up quickly.

The child with a true pulp space infection has a throbbing finger that probably "kept him or her awake last night" and that the child may be holding high to ease the pain. Redness, swelling, and marked tenderness of the distal pulp space will be present, although fluctuation will not be evident because the compartments are small.

Surgical drainage is required and should be carried out, usually under general anesthesia, as soon as the diagnosis can be made with confidence. The traditional sites for incision along each side of the terminal digit were formerly used for the insertion of through-and-through drains. Most physicians now believe satisfactory drainage can be achieved through the site where the abscess most closely approaches the surface, with effort taken to avoid the prime touch surface so far as is possible.

Drainage is customarily achieved under antibiotic coverage. However, as with other infections requiring surgical care, the decision regarding antibiotic therapy should not influence when and how drainage is obtained.

Herpetic Whitlow

Infection of the fingertip with the herpesvirus is fairly common and usually occurs in the young child or infant who also has a herpetic labialis or stomatitis. The fingertip may be red and swollen, simulating a bacterial felon; the diagnosis is evident when one notes small blisters on the surface filled with water-clear liquid. There will be some tenderness but not as much as one would expect with a bacterial infection. If electron microscopy is available on an emergency basis, the diagnosis can be confirmed within minutes by examination of the liquid, which will contain the viral bodies.

The course of this lesion is one of gradual resolution, and it is controversial whether drainage and debridement of the blisters speed the process.

Purulent Tenosynovitis

Although there is little difference in purulent tenosynovitis when seen in children from its presentation in adults, its serious nature and the need for early diagnosis justify its inclusion here.

The flexor tendons to each of the middle three fingers lie within a sheath that extends from the level of the distal interphalangeal joint up to the level of the metacarpophalangeal joint. The flexor sheaths for the thumb and little finger extend proximally to the wrist level where they communicate. Because of this, tenosynovitis of one of the central fingers remains localized to that finger, whereas such an infection involving either the thumb or the little finger may spread proximally to the wrist level and then back distally into the sheath of the communicating but previously uninvolved digit.

Most cases of purulent tenosynovitis are due to direct contamination from the exterior by a puncture wound. The usual causative organism is either *Staphylococcus* or *Streptococcus*.

Inspection reveals the involved finger to be (1) swollen, particularly on the palmar aspect, and (2) held in slight flexion. There will be (3) tenderness over the extent of the tendon sheath, and (4) severe pain will be produced by even slight passive extension of the finger. These are Kanavel's four cardinal signs of suppurative tenosynovitis.

Urgent referral for surgical care is required whenever bacterial tenosynovitis is suspected. Prompt drainage and irrigation of the sheath plus systemic antibiotic therapy are required and must be instituted without delay if there is to be any hope for ultimate normal tendon function.

Palmar Space Infections

Thenar and mid-palmar space infections are uncommon, but when these infections are seen experienced surgical judgment for the decisions regarding diagnosis and drainage is required. The thenar space lies fairly superficially, anterior to the adductor pollicis muscle, over the more medial part of the thenar eminence. The mid-palmar space is situated deep in the central palm, beneath the flexor tendons, which run to the middle, ring, and little fingers.

Infection in either of the palmar spaces produces the expected swelling, redness, tenderness, and possibly fluctuation over the site of the involved space. Interestingly, edema over the dorsum of the hand is also noted. Although this edema may be even more marked than in the palm, this should not distract attention from the offending aspect of the hand.

Drainage under antibiotic cover is the recommended treatment and should be embarked on without delay.

Lymphangitis and Lymphadenitis

Spread of bacterial infection by way of lymphatic channels produces red streaking up the limb (lymphangitis) and inflammation of the regional lymph nodes (lymphadenitis). Infections that show early lymphatic spread are likely to be due to *Streptococcus*. This organism elaborates hyaluronidase, which acts to inhibit clotting and hence encourages lymphatic dissemination. Pyogenic staphylococci, on the other hand, produce coagulase, which induces fibrin clotting and, therefore, favors confinement of the infection. This is the basis for abscess formation. However, lymphangitis can also result from pure staphylococcal infections, mixed staphylococcal and streptococcal infections, or a variety of others, indicating that the bacteriologic diagnosis must remain presumptive until the organism can be cultured.

Although early streaking a few centimeters above the primary infection is usually handled easily with oral antibiotic therapy on an outpatient basis, established lymphangitis extending halfway up an extremity is indication for aggressive intravenous antibacterial therapy as an inpatient. With the appropriate agent, rapid response can be expected and the systemic complications such as septicemia or bacterial endocarditis, so feared in the preantibiotic era, should not be a problem in the previously healthy child.

Axillary or inguinal adenitis may occur when infection in the primary site is still evident. Conversely, it may not appear until days after the primary site appears to have healed completely. For this reason, it is quite common for one not to be able to find the primary infection site.

Antibiotic therapy using a drug appropriate for gram-positive organisms is indicated and will, in all likelihood, induce resolution in short order. However, the mass will on occasion enlarge, demonstrate increasing inflammatory reaction, and perhaps even fluctuate. Surgical drainage is then necessary. Long courses of a variety of antibiotics in the hope of preventing the need for surgical drainage do little other than prolong the course of the illness. Once the initial response to antibiotic therapy is seen to be inadequate and abscess formation is apparent, discontinuation of the antibiotic will permit the abscess to mature and come to drainage sooner. On the other hand, systemic toxicity from the infection and underlying disease, such as congenital heart disease, are indications for persisting with antibiotic treatment even after the need for surgical drainage is noted.

Cat-Scratch Adenitis

A specific form of lymphadenitis occurs from time to time after a scratch, less often after a bite, from a cat. Initially a small papule appears at the site of the scratch within a few days. This is often unnoticed, and there may be no remaining cutaneous manifestations of the initial scratch when, several weeks later, acute lymphadenitis develops. Since most cat scratches are on the hands or forearms, the axillary nodes are most often involved. The nodes are very tender, sometimes markedly enlarged, but do not often develop into one discrete fluctuant mass. The adenitis customarily resolves gradually after a number of weeks, with no residual abnormality.

When the nodes do fluctuate, as they will in the occasional instance, aspiration or incisional drainage reveals liquid, which grows nothing on routine bacteriology. Although a recently isolated microorganism is considered as a good possibility, the etiologic agent has not, as yet, been identified. The axillary mass will remain for a number of weeks with or without drainage, but eventual complete resolution can be expected.

Infections of Bone and Joint

Acute Hematogenous Osteomyelitis

Bacterial infection in bone is far from a daily occurrence even in a busy pediatric emergency department. However, its potential for leading to serious systemic infection, the risk of permanent deformity, and the tendency to be the precursor of a chronic state that may last for years in spite of the best treatment are all strong indicators of the importance of this serious disease and the necessity for prompt recognition and experienced management.

In most instances, acute hematogenous osteomyelitis begins in the metaphysis of a long bone, close to the epiphyseal plate, where the capillaries demonstrate sharply angled hairpin bends and are the site of lodgment of small bacterial emboli. Decreased numbers of macrophages have also been reported in this location and may further predispose to progression of infection. Local abscess formation creates an area of pressure because of the edema and increased vascular supply to the area. The infection spreads to and through the cortex as the pressure it produces compromises blood supply to the immediately adjacent bone and results in necrosis of that portion of bone. When the cortex has been penetrated, the periosteum becomes separated from the bone, permitting the pus to spread up and down until the point is reached at which the periosteum remains tightly attached to the bone, at the epiphyseal plate. Hence, the exudate readily extends down the bone as it lifts up the periosteum but is stopped at the epiphyseal plate. If the elevation of the periosteum is extensive, the underlying cortical bone is deprived also of its periosteal blood supply and dies, becoming a sequestrum. In addition, the elevated periosteum lays down a tube of new bone in its elevated position. This is the involucrum. Radiographic demonstration of even the first indication of sequestrum and involucrum establishes that the disease has progressed to its chronic stage.

Most cases of hematogenous osteomyelitis are due to pyogenic staphylococci. There are other organisms cultured on occasion, although it is sometimes difficult to rule out superinfection in such cases. In the debilitated child with septicemia, almost any organism may seed out into bone at a number of sites. Bone infections due to direct external contamination may be caused by a variety of organisms, including *Pseudomonas*. Tuberculous osteomyelitis has become exceedingly rare in pediatric practice in the developed world.

Complications that may occur during the course of acute hematogenous osteomyelitis include acute cellulitis over the site of the subperiosteal abscess; septicemia and pyemic abscesses; septic arthritis due to intra-articular extension; and progression to the chronic stage with sequestra and draining sinuses, pathologic fracture and bony deformity, and growth disturbance.

The clinical picture in cases of acute osteomyelitis of a long bone is usually quite characteristic. Steady pain rapidly becoming severe that is located near the end of a long bone should immediately merit consideration as an acute bone infection. The presence of a history of trauma should not remove totally the suspicion of infection because there is a history of mild trauma prior to the onset of the osteomyelitis in many instances. This may be merely because one would be hard-put to find a day in which an active child has not had some sort of traumatic episode. Alternatively, it may be that trauma to an extremity results in a small hematoma within the bone that becomes infected.

Within a matter of hours to a day, the pain becomes unbearable. Overlying tenderness and, as time passes, edema become apparent. Subsequently systemic manifestations, such as fever and leukocytosis, can be expected, although changes in temperature or white cell count are not sufficiently consistent to be of great diagnostic value.

Fortunately few children demonstrate progression of disease beyond this stage because prompt treatment is usually effective at stopping the progression. However, prior to the era of antibiotic therapy, the high fever and delirium of septicemia were observed to occur in an alarming number of cases.

Osteomyelitis also occurs in the neonatal period and early infancy, with devastating results. Although pain and swelling occur, they are difficult to recognize in early infancy. All too often systemic manifestations such as fever are absent in the small baby. Hence, it is even more important in the young infant to keep bone and joint infection in mind because the diagnosis is often seriously delayed.

Radiographic changes do not occur until at least 6 or 7 days after the onset of the disease in the small baby and from 8 to 10 days in the older child. Therefore, radiography is of little value at the very time one would wish it to be of help in confirming the diagnosis. The diagnosis of osteomyelitis in its early stages remains clinical and must be kept in mind whenever pain in a long bone is not clearly explained on the basis of trauma. Orthopaedic consultation should be sought liberally in such situations because of the serious consequences of diagnostic delay.

Although children with suspected osteomyelitis should be under the care of an orthopaedic surgeon, initial steps in management should be begun before the surgeon has arrived. In addition to routine blood work, several samples should be sent for blood culture and bacterial sensitivity. Routine urinalysis as well as other requirements for preanesthetic work-up should be carried out. A venous infusion should be established as a vehicle for antibiotic administration. For the early case, the initiation of antibacterial therapy may be deferred until the orthopaedic surgeon has arrived and concurs. On the other hand, if the orthopaedic surgeon's arrival will be delayed, or if the child is particularly ill, high-dose treatment using an antistaphylococcal agent, such as cloxacillin or one of the later-generation cephalosporins, should be started at once.

If begun in time, intravenous antibiotic therapy using an appropriate drug in the appropriately high dosage will result in complete resolution of the symptoms in a few days. The medication should be continued for weeks, however, because it has been shown that this is necessary to minimize subsequent flare-ups. Careful orthopaedic observation during the first few hours is essential because drainage will be necessary if there is not marked and rapid improvement on medical therapy.

Acute Septic Arthritis

Background material necessary to a discussion of septic arthritis is presented in Chapter 34. Although bacterial infection of the hip joint is the most common form of joint sepsis in children, other joints are occasionally involved. The clinical presentation is one of pain that is worse with movement, effusion, and marked limitation of passive movement. Systemic manifestations of infection will vary in severity from slight fever to the clinical picture of septicemia.

Septic arthritis, like osteomyelitis, can be extremely difficult to diagnose in early infancy. Any baby who is irritable, even slightly febrile, and not using all four limbs normally should be considered as having septic arthritis, osteomyelitis, or both until one can be confident otherwise.

In the majority of instances, joint sepsis is due to *Staphylococcus aureus*. Other organisms that have been cultured include *Haemophilus influenzae*, *Streptococcus hemolyticus*, *Streptococcus pneumoniae*, *Salmonella*, *Brucella*, and *Neisseria gonorrhoeae*. For practical purposes, tuberculous arthritis has been eliminated from pediatric practice in developed countries.

Articular cartilage is quickly and readily destroyed by joint sepsis. Consequently, there is particular urgency in the diagnosis of and initiation of treatment for bacterial joint infection. This applies especially in early infancy, when the presentation can be so indefinite. Referral to an orthopaedist for appropriate antibiotic therapy and surgical drainage must not be delayed for even an hour.

37

Osteochondroses

General Considerations

Osteochondroses are a group of epiphyseal lesions with ischemic necrosis as the basic initiating process, a series of histopathologic changes common to all, and varied clinical presentations that depend on the age of the child and the site of the epiphysis involved. Most examples of osteochondrosis, whatever the anatomic site, are referred to clinic or office for orthopaedic consultation and are not seen in the emergency department. However, at some stage pain is a feature of these conditions, and the occasional child with osteochondrosis will arrive in the emergency department with as yet undiagnosed pain or pain that is unexpectedly more severe than usual. Hence, the emergency physician should be aware of osteochondroses, although this chapter does not discuss osteochondroses in the detail one would see in an orthopaedic presentation.

One can conveniently classify osteochondroses into three main groups, which are dependent on the types of epiphyses involved:

1. Those that involve secondary centers of ossification that are generally weight bearing and contribute to bone length.
2. Those that involve primary centers of ossification. These are usually in small bones that have no secondary centers and, since they are largely covered with cartilage, have a rather precarious blood supply at best.
3. Those that involve traction epiphyses (apophyses). Current orthopaedic teaching suggests that in most of these, repetitive trauma plays a part in etiology. This sets traction epiphyses apart from the other osteochondroses for which etiology is for the most part unknown.

In spite of the apparent differences among the groups of osteochondroses, the anatomic and radiographic changes that the bones undergo during the course of the disease are markedly similar in all cases. There are four basic stages in the pathologic process that have been described and that correspond to recognized radiographic changes. These stages merge one with the other, and each may occupy a number of years of the child's life before proceeding to completion. The sequence of these stages follows:

1. *Avascularity.*   This is the phase of ischemic bone death that is usually asymptomatic. The avascular bone remains unchanged, although the cells have died. Because it has stopped growing, the epiphysis becomes relatively smaller than the contralateral epiphysis. As articular cartilage is nourished by the synovial fluid and not by blood vessels, it remains viable and continues to grow. Therefore, the cartilage space thickens, as seen on x-ray film.

2. *Revascularization.*   Ingrowing blood vessels permit new bone growth that occurs around the bony infarct, producing increased density on x-ray film. The new bone is of normal bony strength and hardness but will mold with external forces and is said to have "biologic plasticity." It is this property which results in deformity. Therapeutic efforts are directed toward influencing external forces to minimize this deformity.

   The combined processes of bony resorption and deposition continue side by side and may take several years to replace the dead bone completely. During this period a subperiosteal fracture is common and may be in large part responsible both for pain (e.g., the discomfort of Legg-Calvé-Perthes disease) and for the degree to which the bone is vulnerable to deforming forces. Some osteochondroses, in particular that of the femoral head, demonstrate subluxation at this stage also, as a result of developing incongruency within the joint.

3. *Bone healing.*   When replacement of the dead bone has finished, resorption stops, but bony deposition continues. The bone is still susceptible to molding forces as it grows.

4. *Residual deformity.*   The amount of deformity that has resulted from the stages of gradual revascularization and bone healing is permanent, and the degree of symptoms that develop later on depends on the degree of this deformity.

Treatment plans depend completely on the natural history of the specific osteochondrosis. For aseptic necrosis of the femoral head, the goal of treatment is to maintain suitable molding forces around the head while it remains plastic. For other osteochondroses, such as the capitellum or the tarsal navicular bone, there is no risk of deformity and treatment need only be symptomatic.

Specific Osteochondroses

Osteochondroses Involving Secondary Centers of Ossification

Femoral Capital Epiphysis (Legg-Calvé-Perthes Disease)

Legg-Calvé-Perthes disease occurs between the ages of 3 and 10, is more common in boys, and usually appears in the revascularization stage of the disease with pain and limp. The pain is in the known distribution of pain caused by hip disease (i.e., anywhere from groin to knee). The limp is classically a Trendelenburg gait but very frequently demonstrates a combination of antalgic and Trendelenburg components.

Many instances of Legg-Calvé-Perthes disease have as their first manifestation of the condition an acute episode, which, to all intents and purposes, is an attack of monarticular synovitis. Hence the need for first-attack cases of synovitis to undergo radiographic evaluation. In instances of recurrent synovitis, Legg-Calvé-Perthes disease must be even more suspect. Therefore, if radiographs remain normal and there is strong reason to rule out Legg-Calvé-Perthes disease, a bone scan may help.

The diagnosis and treatment decisions required in osteochondrosis of the femoral head require experienced orthopaedic care.

Capitellum (Panner's Disease)

Panner's disease is a rare condition that affects children between the ages of 3 and 11. The elbow is not a weight-bearing joint, and there is little chance of deformity developing as the ischemic capitellum reossifies. Hence, treatment is symptomatic only, and the prognosis is excellent.

Metatarsal Head (Freiberg's Disease)

Usually involving the head of the second or, less commonly, the third metatarsal of an adolescent girl, Freiberg's disease can be of very significant nuisance value and may require special shoe appliances to minimize pain. Ultimately excision of the metatarsal head may be required.

Thoracic Spine (Scheuermann's Disease)

Dull mid-thoracic spinal pain and developing kyphosis in an adolescent boy or girl are characteristic of Scheuermann's disease. The diagnosis is radiographic. The treatment, aimed at preventing deformity, necessitates experienced orthopaedic judgment.

Osteochondroses Involving Primary Centers of Ossification

Tarsal Navicular Bone (Köhler's Disease)

Low-grade pain, limp, and tenderness over the area of the navicular bone in a 4- to 8-year-old child (more commonly a boy) all suggest Köhler's disease, which is confirmed radiographically. Treatment is symptomatic, and the ultimate prognosis is excellent.

Vertebral Body (Calvé's Syndrome)

In the 2- to 8-year-old child, ill-defined back pain, possibly mild paraspinal spasm, and a slight kyphosis may lead to radiographs of the spine on which necrosis of one vertebral body is seen. There is evidence that at least some of these cases are due to a localized intravertebral eosinophilic granuloma that has squashed with the forces of body weight. Orthopaedic referral is required.

Osteochondroses Involving Traction Epiphyses (Post-Traumatic Apophysitis)

Tibial Tuberosity (Osgoode-Schlatter Disease)

A history of pain and soreness over the tibial tuberosity, with visible swelling, tenderness, and pain on extension against resistance, all serve to establish the diagnosis of Osgoode-Schlatter disease. Radiographs are not always required but show soft tissue edema and apophyseal fragmentation when obtained. This condition is frequently bilateral, although it may start on the second leg months after the first. Treatment, again, is largely symptomatic with activity restriction as required. The outcome is excellent.

Calcaneal Apophysis (Sever's Disease)

Sever's disease is seen in particularly active children between 8 and 15 years of age. Pain at the heel cord attachment during the take-off phase of walking or running and slight swelling with tenderness over this site are the diagnostic criteria. There is a wide range of normal in the radiographs of this apophysis, so radiographs are usually of little help. Although it may last a year or so, this condition is self-limited. Treatment is symptomatic and designed to decrease the traction on the calcaneal apophysis when the calf muscles contract. A 1-cm lift in the heel of the shoe helps.

Musculoskeletal Trauma to the Extremities

Soft Tissue Injury

Differentiation from Fracture

In children, ligaments, tendons, and other soft tissues are stronger in relation to bones or epiphyses than they are in adults. This is based on the observation that the incidence of fractures in relation to the incidence of sprains, strains, and other soft tissue injuries is much greater in children than in adults. The younger the child is, the more true this is. Although a damaged knee ligament is sometimes seen in the 10-year-old skier and a sprained ankle is sometimes seen in the 12-year-old ballet dancer, these injuries are distinctly unusual. Even in the teenager, if the epiphyses are still open, one must expect to find and one should first look particularly for fracture or epiphyseal injury. The 11-year-old football player whose knee shows a marked valgus deformity following a blow from the lateral side is more likely to have a fracture-separation at either the lower femoral or the upper tibial epiphysis than a disrupted ligament. Similarly, the 9-year-old who has turned the ankle and has tenderness over it laterally is more likely to have a fracture-separation of the lower fibular epiphysis than the sprain one would expect after the epiphyses have closed.

The diagnosis, "soft tissue injury," valid so often in the adult population, should be applied sparingly in children. Too often this diagnosis is applied to the child whose fracture is obscure and remains undetected because the physician forgets that children experience fractures in preference to soft tissue injuries and does not put enough effort into finding it. "Pulled muscle" is another diagnosis used too freely in children. Avulsion of an apophysis, or some other form of an epiphyseal injury, is more likely. Important diagnoses may be missed with serious consequences on the grounds that all that is wrong is a pulled muscle.

Only when fracture or epiphyseal fracture-separation has been looked for carefully should one accept the diagnosis of sprain, strain, or soft tissue injury.

Contusions

Severe muscular contusions require active treatment. At first, repeated icing of the injured area and compression bandage may slow or stop the bleeding. Active exercise combined with various physiotherapeutic modalities accelerate the return to full function, although severe muscular contusions can cause relative disability for some time and are of particular importance to competing athletes. Aspiration or surgical drainage of intramuscular hematomas is rarely required. Rarely the edema and hemorrhage of a severe muscle contusion may result in a compartment syndrome, in which the pressure increase within the fascial compartment can seriously compromise vascular inflow. Fasciotomy is required for an established compartment syndrome.

Minor bruises are seen by every physician and are of nuisance value only. However, there is a question that needs to be asked whenever a contusion on an extremity is encountered: is there enough suspicion of an underlying fracture to indicate radiographic examination? This is often a difficult question, and many radiographs are taken of bruised extremities because the examiner cannot make the differentiation on clinical grounds alone. Frequently, these radiographs are unnecessary.

Although tenderness is characteristic of both contusion and fracture, it is usually possible to make the differentiation between the two on physical examination only. If there is a fracture, the application of indirect stress to the bone, which may be longitudinal compression, twisting, or bending, without touching the tender site directly, should elicit pain. None of these stresses should generate pain with a contusion.

Careful examination of the extremity that has sustained direct trauma is one way, perhaps the most practical way, to minimize unnecessary extremity radiographs.

General Aspects of Extremity Fractures

Etiology

Pediatric fractures are common and are caused by a limitless variety of traumatic situations. In most instances, a single major traumatic episode can be described. Less often several episodes of violence are described, the last of which is the likely culprit. A stress fracture, usually involving one of the bones of the foot, is produced by repeated minor traumas.

The vast majority of fractures are sustained in previously normal, strong bones. However, pathologic fractures do occur through single bony lesions, such as a unicameral bone cyst, or through diffuse bony abnormalities. Examples of this would be regional osteoporosis in the lower limb bones of a child who is paraplegic because of spina bifida and generalized brittleness of osteogenesis imperfecta.

A situation frequently serving as the clue to abuse is fracture of a long bone in the young child. Nonaccidental external violence causes a significant proportion of long bone fractures in the young child and should be kept in mind for consideration in all. In the child who has been subjected to physical abuse, radiographic investigation frequently demonstrates multiple fractures of rib cage, skull, and extremities, with the fractures showing various stages of union in different sites. For this reason, a basic skeletal series is usually part of the general work-up of a suspected abuse case.

Different Forms of Pediatric Fractures

In the common greenstick fracture, bending of the bone occurs with breaking only on its convex side and is analogous to the bending with partial breaking only of a green stick which one tries to break over one's knee.

The "buckle" or torus fracture is usually seen near the ends of long bones and in some ways is a form of a greenstick fracture. In a buckle fracture, the bone usually bends but does not break along the convex side of the fracture and buckles along the concave side. This produces a small wrinkle or angulation inward on the surface of the bone often visible only on the lateral radiograph. It is likely that the child sent home by the inexperienced physician with the diagnosis "soft tissue injury to wrist" has a buckle fracture of the distal radius, which may be evident on close perusal of the lateral projection.

An uncommon form of fracture seen in the more bendable pediatric long bone is the "bowing" fracture, in which the radiograph demonstrates a curve in the shaft resulting from a myriad of tiny microfractures. Not only is experienced judgment necessary to decide if the degree of bowing requires reduction, but also an experienced hand is needed to achieve satisfactory reduction, which can be very difficult in the bowing fracture.

Radiographic Diagnosis

Many fractures in infancy and early childhood are difficult to visualize radiographically. Buckle fractures can be so obscure as to be undetectable even to the examiner who suspects and looks for the buckle.

A hairline crack in a toddler's tibia can sometimes be seen only on special views. The presence of some toddlers' tibial fractures and of some undisplaced supracondylar elbow fractures cannot be established by usual radiographic techniques until new bone is visible on the film obtained 10 days later. In these situations, one learns that the clinical findings are of the utmost importance. The child whom the careful clinician thinks has a buckle fracture of the radius probably does.

Soft tissue shadows may be useful aids in interpreting the radiographs. The 2-year-old whose injured elbow just demonstrates an effusion on radiograph probably has the supracondylar fracture that the physician was looking for.

The radiographs of most infant joints are difficult to interpret. When the radiograph of the fractured elbow of an infant is examined, much information must be derived by inference alone. The bulk of the joint structure is still cartilaginous in infancy and is therefore radiolucent. Hence, the configuration of a fracture, to a large extent, must be inferred from the position of any epiphyses which already show some early calcification and from the portion of the fracture line visibly extending into the metaphysis.

Avoiding the Missed Fracture

However, from time to time important radiographic diagnoses in infancy and childhood are missed on first visit with undesirable consequences. Failure to recognize a significant extremity fracture is often blamed either on neglecting to obtain a radiograph or on inadequacies in interpreting the radiograph. With very few exceptions, such outcomes result from either of two things: failure to examine the patient carefully enough or failure to think of and look for serious injury. When the physician has identified the site of the lesion through careful examination, when he or she knows what conditions occur most commonly in children, when he or she is attuned to looking for the most serious possibility, and when he or she has requested only the appropriate radiographs, the likelihood of missing a fracture is minimal.

Types of Deformity in Pediatric Fractures

The main forms of radiologic deformity of a fractured long bone, namely displacement, shortening, rotation, and angulation, are the same for children as for adults. However, the need to correct a certain deformity in the management of a child's fracture may be vastly different from the need to correct that same deformity in an adult extremity.

Children have remarkable powers to remold and obliterate a deformity that is pure displacement, and the younger the child is, the greater is the degree of displacement which can be accepted. This knowledge is useful when deciding which fractures need to be reduced as well as during the management of fractures in which difficulty is encountered in obtaining anatomic reduction.

Shortening in an adult femur or tibia produces permanent leg length discrepancy. In a child, one may even desire a fractured femur to unite with 1 or 2 cm of overriding and shortening because growth usually accelerates after a fracture as a result of the increased blood supply required for the healing process and its stimulant effect on the epiphyses.

Rotation is not particularly age dependent, and for practical purposes, the same degrees of rotation that need to be corrected in adults require reduction in children.

Angulation, for the most part, also needs to be corrected. However, the young child will, in time, correct a small amount of angulation if it occurs near a hinge joint and is in the same plane as the plane of movement of that joint. As a result, a few degrees of extension deformity of a distal radial fracture that would need to be corrected in an adult can be accepted in a child because the fracture is close to the wrist joint and the angulation is in the same plane as the flexion-extension movement of the wrist.

Treatment

Plaster immobilization is standard care for most pediatric fractures, whether the cast is applied after reduction of a displaced fracture or for management of one that requires no reduction. The cast must be carefully molded so that it has a snug grip on and has the same shape as the contained limb. The distal forearm is not circular in cross section but oval, and the cast should reflect that configuration. The elbow is usually best held at 90 degrees of flexion and to maintain that position the cast must be sharply molded around the olecranon. Too often the above-elbow cast displays a gentle curve as it passes over the back of the elbow, thus permitting the arm to slip up and down in it.

The decision to extend a cast to the axilla or groin as opposed to incorporating only forearm or lower leg varies with the type of fracture, how unstable it is, whether rotation is likely to occur at the fracture site, and how vigorous the child's activities are expected to be during the period of immobilization. Most buckle fractures of the radius are quite stable and are satisfactorily treated in a forearm cast. The real purpose of most such casts is merely to eliminate pain. However, if there is a significant degree of dorsal tilt of the fragment and severe discomfort on pronation or supination, one can infer some risk of increasing deformity unless supination is prevented by a well-molded above-elbow cast. If one does not wish a young child to bear weight on the cast used for a tibial fracture, one may choose to apply it with the knee flexed to 90 percent, thus making it difficult for the child to get the foot on the ground.

The duration of immobilization also varies from fracture to fracture and child to child. The fractured femur of a neonate will be healed solidly in 3 or 4 weeks, but union will take 8 or 9 weeks in the 5-year-old. Buckle fractures of the forearm are usually solid in 3 weeks, whereas displaced shaft fractures of the forearm usually require 6 weeks in plaster after reduction. The supracondylar elbow fracture is well united within 3 weeks, and active movement is necessary from that time on to facilitate return of function and avoid permanent elbow stiffness.

Internal Fixation

Open reduction and internal fixation of closed fractures is reserved for specific situations and is less often indicated in children than in adults. The forearm fracture involving both bones, customarily handled operatively in adults, rarely requires internal fixation in children, in whom a greater degree of displacement can and should be accepted. Femoral shaft fractures treated in traction invariably heal strongly in otherwise healthy children and require no surgical intervention. On the other hand, intramedullary nailing of a femoral shaft fracture may be indicated to facilitate nursing care in the child who is restless and thrashing about because of a head injury. Modern developments in fracture care in children have led to operative fixation for some fractures that formerly were always treated nonoperatively. Pin fixation of the displaced supracondylar fracture of the humerus following reduction is an example. Internal fixation removes the need for the undesirable and risky nonphysiologic position necessary when plaster immobilization was the treatment of choice and, consequently, has reduced the risk of vascular complications.

Open Fractures

Open fractures require aggressive surgical care. Too often a fracture that has a small puncture wound as the only indication of the open nature of the injury is treated with minimal debridement and primary closure under local anesthesia. This form of management is fraught with danger and is just the type of situation that puts the patient at risk for serious infection, even clostridial myositis or gas gangrene. Whenever there is a break in the skin covering the site of a fracture, careful orthopaedic judgment is necessary to decide on the extent of surgical exploration and debridement required.

Epiphysis

General Considerations

Growth in length of long bones is peculiar to the pediatric age group and is made possible by the cartilaginous growth plate, or epiphyseal plate, near the end of the bone, both ends in most instances. Because presence of the epiphysis and of the growth plate itself is characteristic of the child, so are the specific types of fractures involving this area. Some epiphyseal fractures jeopardize future growth of the affected bone. Many others do not. The need to recognize the type of epiphyseal fracture and its prognosis and to select the appropriate treatment is an important feature of pediatric trauma practice. An understanding of the injuries and their prognosis requires a basic knowledge of the histologic anatomy of the epiphyseal plate itself (Fig. 38–1).

The layer of the cartilage plate nearest the end of the bone contains proliferating cartilage cells that line up in parallel rows as they divide, adding length to the bone. The adjacent layer moves distally along with the zone of proliferating cells, keeping the proliferating zone a constant width. This second layer is produced by calcification of the cartilaginous intercellular substance, a process which results in death of the cartilage cells because it prevents diffusion, the mechanism by which cartilage cells are nourished. This dead layer, or the layer of provisional calcification, is then "attacked" by osteoclasts, which ingest the debris. Accompanied by blood vessels, undifferentiated cells invade from the proximal side of the plate, differentiate into osteoblasts, and lay down the intercellular substance of bone.

In essence, the layer of provisional calcification is formed adjacent to the growing cartilage layer as intercellular substance calcifies. It is removed at the other side where osteoclasts eliminate it and new bone is formed. Hence, this zone of provisional calcification remains a constant thickness while, at the same time, moving distally along with the zone of proliferating cartilage cells. Epiphyseal fracture-separations usually occur within the zone of provisional calcification, the "dead zone," or at its junction with the zone of proliferation and therefore do not put the proliferating cartilage cells, or bone growth, at risk, provided that the fracture does not deviate toward the proliferating layer. However, because the fracture crosses the bone through radiolucent cartilage, it is not visible on the radiograph, unless it deviates into bone.

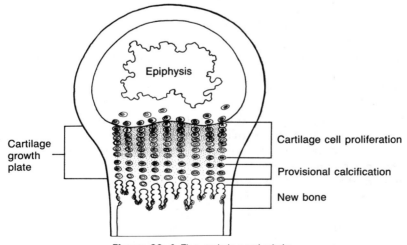

Figure 38–1 The epiphyseal plate.

Epiphyseal fractures have been classified into five basic groups, which are determined by the configuration of the fracture itself (Harris-Salter classification). The treatment required for a specific injury and its prognosis depend largely on a recognition of the category into which the example fits.

Epiphyseal Fracture-Separations: The Harris-Salter Classification (Fig. 38-2)

Type I. A type I fracture passes completely across the plate, without straying either proximally or distally. Classically this injury is produced by a longitudinal pull. The most common example is the fracture of the lower fibular epiphysis seen when a child forcibly inverts the ankle. There is little of note to be seen radiographically except for soft tissue swelling over the lateral malleolus. Radiographic widening of the epiphyseal plate is rare. Although the zone of proliferating cartilage accompanies the epiphysis when this separation occurs and the direction of growth will depend on the ultimate alignment of the epiphysis, there is rarely any significant displacement, nor is there any real risk to growth.

Type II. A type II injury is characterized by a fracture line that crosses the plate part way then deviates into the metaphysis, where it is visible on the radiograph. This means that the distal fracture fragment consists of the epiphysis with a triangular metaphyseal fragment attached to it. Often the fracture line outlining a triangle of metaphysis is the only radiographic clue to the presence of a type II injury. The type II fracture is classically caused by a shearing stress. The periosteum is tough and thick in children, and as the epiphysis is shoved off the bone by the shearing force it is held against the metaphysis by this strong periosteal tube. Hence, it is pulled proximally as it shears and takes a metaphyseal triangle with it. In a pure type II injury there should be no growth disturbance because, as in the type I fracture, the fracture line does not approach the zone of proliferating cartilage. However, the growing cartilage moves with the epiphyseal fragment, and malaligned growth will occur if there is significant displacement. Reduction is usually easy, though, and normal growth can be anticipated after union. An exception to this absence of growth disturbance with type II injury occurs when there has been an unexpected component of the mechanical force directed longitudinally, producing compression of the plate at the same time (type V). Although rare, this can be manifest in a growth disturbance at some site in the plate which may become apparent weeks or months after the trauma.

Type III. In the type III injury, the fracture line crosses part of the plate and then turns toward the end of the bone, crossing the zone of proliferating cartilage cells in doing so, and leaves the bone after traversing the epiphysis itself. The classic example of this injury is the Tillaux fracture. This occurs in the girl who is usually 12 or 13 years old or in the boy several years older. At this age the lower tibial epiphyseal plate is closing. This is a gradual process and occurs from the medial side to the lateral. Consequently there is an appreciable period, a number of months, during which the medial portion of the epiphyseal plate is solidly fused and the lateral portion is still open. In this situation longitudinal compression force or torsion can break the still open part of the plate. When this happens, the laterally situated epiphyseal fragment breaks free from the medial portion. If this form of epiphyseal fracture were seen in the younger child, there would be significant potential damage to the growing cartilage. In the 13-year-old girl or 15-year-old boy, it is the state of partial closure of the epiphysis that puts the bone at risk for this injury, and at this stage, needless to say, growth has finished. Examples of this injury elsewhere in the body can occur before closure has begun but fortunately are uncommon. In these, risk of growth disturbance is somewhat reduced by achieving and maintaining accurate reduction.

Type IV. The fracture line of a type IV injury crosses epiphysis, plate, and metaphysis so that the fracture fragment consists of portions of epiphysis, plate, and metaphysis. Accurate reduction is neces-

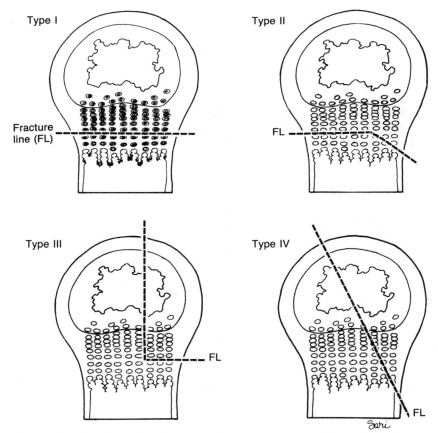

Figure 38–2 Epiphyseal fracture types I through IV. In types I, II, and III, the fracture line (FL) follows the zone of provisional calcification for all or part of the way. In type IV, the FL crosses epiphysis, plate, and metaphysis.

sary in a type IV injury to prevent growth disturbance. Even slight proximal displacement of the fragment can result in cross union between the epiphyseal portion of the fragment and the metaphysis, effectively preventing further growth at that location. Cessation of growth and deformed growth can be the outcome. This is of particular significance in the lower extremity, where length discrepancies can be so disabling. These injuries require orthopaedic attention.

Type V. In the type V injury, crush damage to the proliferating cartilage cells results in slowed or uneven growth leading to deformity. One may only guess that a child has sustained a type V injury when seen initially. However, when a child has sustained a vague ankle injury after jumping from the garage roof but no fracture or other clear diagnosis can be made, the possibility of a type V injury that might show up weeks or months later must be entertained. Type V injuries may be isolated but can also be produced in combination with other forms of epiphyseal trauma. A type II fracture-separation of a distal radial epiphysis may unite solidly and quickly, but growth disturbance may begin to appear months later on the basis of a type V compression injury sustained at the same time.

Attempts should be made to assign a classification to each epiphyseal fracture seen. This serves very effectively as the basis on which the risk of growth disturbance following an epiphyseal injury can be estimated. Union of an epiphyseal fracture-separation is rapid, and the duration of necessary immobilization is roughly one-half that required for a fracture of the shaft of the same bone. Some epiphyseal fractures, particularly those involving smaller bones, may be solidly united within 2 weeks. This is an advantage in most instances but also means that an epiphyseal injury brought for treatment several days after it occurred can be so solidly stuck that closed reduction may be impossible.

Apophysis

An apophysis is an epiphysis which does not contribute to growth in length of the bone and is the site of attachment of a ligament or tendon. Examples of these are the tibial tuberosity, olecranon, coronoid process, and medial epicondyle of the elbow and around the hip either of the trochanters or either of the anterior iliac spines. An apophyseal plate has the same histologic structure as the epiphyseal plate, and it fuses at approximately the same time as the long bone epiphyses are closing. However, the only type of apophyseal fracture that occurs with any frequency is avulsion, resulting in a type I separation. Some apophyseal avulsions necessitate open reduction and internal fixation, such as the displaced medial epicondyle of the elbow. Others are treated nonoperatively, such as the avulsed anterior inferior iliac spine.

Upper Extremity Injuries

Fractures of the Clavicle

The clavicle is easily and frequently broken. This injury is seen most often in the child between 1 and 4 years of age; however, it does occur at all ages, from the neonate whose collarbone is broken by an exceptionally vigorous obstetrician's finger to the 15-year-old hockey player who crashes into the boards. Except in the neonate, most clavicles are broken when the child falls, landing on the shoulder.

In most instances, the diagnosis is obvious on clinical grounds alone. Swelling and tenderness over mid-clavicle are evident, and there may be a visible prominence due to bony deformity. The radiographs used are two views, one a straight anteroposterior and the other an upshoot in lieu of a lateral.

A majority of clavicular fractures are of the greenstick variety and are located near mid-shaft. These are usually quite stable and necessitate no treatment beyond a sling for comfort and restriction of activity for 4 or 5 weeks.

When there is a complete fracture with displacement, the fragments tend to override a little. When this is encountered, holding the shoulders back by means of a figure-of-eight bandage has been thought to prevent further overriding and to alleviate pain. Sometimes, however, regardless of the expertness of the application, a figure-of-eight bandage seems to do nothing but make the pain worse. In these instances, we need to realize that the bandage probably does not change the outcome one bit and that it should not be considered mandatory. There is no need to strive for anatomic reduction of the fracture because molding will in time result in a normal configuration, regardless of the initial degree of displacement. Furthermore, the figure-of-eight bandage will not reduce the deformity anyway. If accurate reduction and maintenance of that reduction were important, open reduction, or at the very least the use of a bulky plaster shoulder spica, would be necessary. Fortunately these measures are both much more than is required.

When a figure-of-eight bandage is used, some physicians choose to recall the child every few days to tighten the bandage. Others prefer to instruct parents how to tighten it on a regular basis. An equally favored method is to apply the bandage initially as tightly as can be tolerated and to secure the ends so that they cannot be tampered with further. It is unlikely that the choice of method makes any difference.

Regardless of the treatment selected, all broken collarbones except the completely stable greenstick fractures will continue to demonstrate movement at the fracture site to some degree for a few days and will, therefore, cause pain for that period. For this reason, analgesia is in order for the first 3 or 4 days after the injury.

Clavicular fractures unite solidly in 3 to 5 weeks, depending on the age of the child, although contact sports should be avoided for another 3 to 5 weeks.

During the process of union of a displaced clavicular fracture, a large lump of bony callus can be expected to develop. Similarly a solid lump over the mid-clavicle may be noted by the parents of a 2- or 3-week-old baby. This lump doubtless represents an unrecognized fracture that was sustained at birth. Parents should be reassured that the callus of a clavicular fracture will gradually disappear over months or years, although a large callus in a teenager may not disappear completely.

In the teenager or young adult, several uncommon types of clavicular fractures require consultation and rarely operation. When there is a central, or "butterfly," fragment that is turned through 90 degrees and is tenting the skin with its pointed end, more aggressive treatment should be considered. Open reduction may be needed to prevent erosion of the skin by the superficial end or of a subclavian vessel by its inner end. When the extreme lateral end of the clavicle is broken off downward, displacement of the terminal fragment along with depression of the shoulder relative to the clavicle indicates rupture of the coracoclavicular ligaments. This is the pediatric analog of the acromioclavicular separation seen in the older patient. Although nonoperative treatment usually suffices, the orthopaedist should make this judgment.

Shoulder Separation

The acromioclavicular separation is rarely seen in individuals under age 15 or 16 because until then the acromioclavicular ligaments are stronger than the end of the clavicle, and they usually pull off a small piece of clavicle instead of rupturing themselves.

Shoulder Dislocation

Dislocations of the shoulder joint are rare in children under the age of 12 years. Although still very uncommon during the early teenage years, shoulder dislocations become more common as time passes.

Forced abduction and external rotation result in a stretch or tear of the anterior capsule, which permits the head to slip out of the glenoid fossa forward and downward. Once this has happened subsequent dislocations occur more easily; the majority seen in any emergency department are recurrences.

The diagnosis is made easily on inspection. A sharp-pointed contour to the shoulder is noted with the lateral aspect dropping straight down from the overhanging acromium because of the absence of the humeral head in the glenoid. Radiographs in at least two projections establish the diagnosis and indicate where the head is actually located.

Neurologic damage, although unusual in the young person, should be looked for. The circumflex nerve particularly should be tested. Significant damage to the elements of the brachial plexus can occur but is more characteristic of the older patient.

Reduction is usually accomplished easily with recurrent dislocations but can be much more difficult when it has never previously occurred. Straight traction in slight abduction with gentle levering of the humeral head out of the axilla is generally quite successful. This can be accomplished either by using the operator's foot against the lateral chest wall just below the axilla or manually by an assistant. It is easy to recognize when reduction occurs because there is a readily felt "clunk," the shape of the shoulder immediately returns to normal, and discomfort is relieved. Postreduction films are warranted after the first episode not so much to establish that the head is back in place but to identify any fractures of the glenoid lip or elsewhere that may have occurred at the same time as the dislocation.

Following reduction, the shoulder should be restricted from external rotation, abduction, or excessive movement in any direction for 4 to 6 weeks. An easy method is to suspend the arm in a sling, which is then bandaged to the patient's chest. The patient must be made well aware of the importance of avoiding external rotation and abduction because the initial discomfort will disappear quickly. The tendency for young people is to return to full and vigorous activity as soon as the pain has gone.

For particularly obese or muscular individuals, reduction can be extremely difficult. In this situation, it may be useful to sedate the youth with intravenous hypnotic and position him or her prone on the stretcher with the affected arm hanging straight down over the side. As muscular relaxation ensues, spontaneous reduction may even occur. If not, relocation of the humeral head can usually be obtained by firm but persistent downward traction on the arm.

Kocher's maneuver, in which the externally rotated arm is briskly internally rotated by swinging the forearm across the patient's chest, is not as free of complications as are the other methods and is recommended only for the experienced.

Each time a shoulder dislocates one can presume more damage has been inflicted on the capsular structures. For this reason, the patient with a shoulder that has a history of recurrent dislocation should be seen orthopaedically for consideration of surgical repair.

For practical purposes, posterior dislocations are not encountered in children.

Upper Humeral Fractures

The epiphyseal plate lies at the level of the anatomic neck of the humerus. Fractures at this level tend to be type II epiphyseal separations, although it is often difficult to visualize the exact morphology of the fracture from the radiograph. Displaced fracture-separations usually need to be reduced in marked flexion and internal rotation (the salute position) and are immobilized in this position for several weeks before the arm can be brought down to the side of the body. This requires orthopaedic consultation. Undisplaced separations, or those very minimally displaced, can usually be handled conveniently in a simple sling for about 3 weeks.

Buckle fractures of the surgical neck are common and unite solidly with sling immobilization for a few weeks.

Humeral Shaft Fractures

Oblique fractures of the shaft of the humerus can damage the radial nerve. Hence, care must be taken to evaluate radial nerve function. Wrist drop and loss of metacarpophalangeal extension should be looked for particularly.

Union is rapid and solid in most instances and does not require absolute immobility. For this reason, a bandage form of splinting is often satisfactory, although a hanging cast and the sugar-tong form of plaster splint are also sometimes preferred. Until early union has ensued, the lower fragment tends to rotate internally, so this must be taken into account when the arm is being immobilized. Orthopaedic advice is in order.

Fracture of the humeral shaft occasionally occurs in the neonate as a result of birth trauma, and radial nerve palsy is an infrequent complication of this injury. In treating a neonatal humeral shaft fracture with radial nerve lesion, it is important to splint the forearm and wrist promptly so the hand cannot fall into flexion, lest the forearm extensor muscles be damaged by this stretching.

Supracondylar Fracture of the Humerus

Although some fractured elbows are caused by falls directly on the elbow, the usual cause is indirect force transmitted up the arm when the child falls on the hand. Either varus or valgus stress can cause a fracture, but such stress is usually combined with posteriorly and longitudinally directed forces. These forces determine the configuration of the fracture and the direction of displacement, if any.

Supracondylar fractures with little or no displacement are common pediatric injuries. In most there is tenderness, swelling, and restricted movement. However, the fairly good range of movement and the minimal tenderness that are occasionally noted can result in the diagnosis being missed entirely.

The radiograph may show very little, although displacement of the anterior and posterior fat pads, indicating an acute hemarthrosis, strongly suggests a fracture with intracapsular extension. When the fracture line is not visible on the initial films, oblique projections of the lower end of the humerus may reveal it. Some undisplaced supracondylar fractures cannot be demonstrated with conventional radiography until new bone becomes apparent along the epicondylar ridges after a week or so.

The undisplaced supracondylar fracture is missed from time to time, resulting in children being discharged with the diagnosis of soft tissue injury or sprain. Failure to make the proper diagnosis is due less often to missing the fracture on the radiograph than failure to remember that in children ligaments and other soft tissues resist damage from trauma longer and more effectively than bones are able to. This means that the child who has injured the elbow by falling on the hand and is thought to have a sprain probably has an undisplaced supracondylar fracture. Remembering this helps to avoid missing the diagnosis.

The child who has the discomfort of a supracondylar fracture, albeit undisplaced, deserves the relief to symptoms provided by a cast. This will permit the child, among other things, to sleep better, without waking up crying every time he or she turns over in bed, striking the elbow. The cast should include the arm from metacarpal heads to axilla, with the elbow at a right angle and the forearm in the mid position. Careful molding of the plaster around the elbow is important. It should be sharply angled around the olecranon to prevent slipping of the cast up and down as time passes. Three weeks in plaster will give time for union and still permit rapid recovery of elbow function.

Displaced supracondylar fractures are characteristic of and virtually unique to children, although much less frequently seen than the undisplaced fractures. They are almost always isolated injuries produced by falls from a height onto the hand. Gross fusiform swelling around the elbow, severe pain, and visible deformity are characteristic. The direction of displacement of the lower humeral fragment is almost always posterior and, in the majority of instances, medial.

This injury has long been associated with a significant incidence of vascular and neurologic damage, and this damage must be sought. A pulseless arm needs prompt reduction of the fracture. If surgical help is not immediately available at the time, gentle traction and slight flexion of the elbow should be attempted in the hope of releasing the brachial artery from the fracture site. If this is not successful, immediate surgical attention will be needed.

Although all three major nerves are in jeopardy with a severely displaced supracondylar fracture, the median nerve is the one most commonly affected. If gross movements of the fingers seem normal, the examiner should check particularly for function of the long flexor of the index finger. The portion of the median nerve that subserves this muscle via the anterior interosseous nerve may be traumatized when there has been no other neurologic damage.

Reduction of a badly displaced supracondylar fracture is a difficult maneuver requiring both experience and meticulous attention.

Although plaster immobilization was the treatment of choice for decades, internal fixation using fine pins is now considered safer and more effective. Internal fixation does not require the markedly flexed position that was necessary when a cast was depended on to maintain reduction and that occasionally further compromised an already borderline vascular supply.

The principle of splinting every fractured limb before radiographs are taken or other procedures are begun is difficult to apply to some supracondylar fractures that are in slight elbow flexion on arrival and may not tolerate any movement. In these instances, laying the child on a stretcher with the arm cradled on a pillow may be the best form of temporary support.

Fractured Lateral Condyle

The type IV fracture-separation of the capitellar portion of the lower humeral epiphysis is a well-recognized pediatric injury, although not as common as the supracondylar fracture. The fracture line begins on the lateral cortex just above the epiphyseal plate, passes medially in the metaphysis to the central portion of the bone, and then turns distally to cross the plate and the epiphysis between the capitellum and trochlea. Type IV separations generally do have the potential for growth disturbance. However, that is distinctly unusual with lateral condylar fractures if good position is maintained, perhaps because the transverse direction of much of the fracture line prevents the proximal displacement that might otherwise result in cross union and subsequent growth abnormality.

Although undisplaced lateral condylar fractures usually unite well with 3 weeks of plaster immobilization with the elbow at 90 degrees, this is a fracture that is fraught with complications, and very intensive follow-up is necessary. Slight displacement can result in nonunion; in others excessive epiphyseal growth can be a late outcome.

The chief indicator of the position of a lateral condylar fracture fragment is the tiny piece of metaphysis that displaces with the capitellum. This is sometimes so tiny as to be almost indiscernible on the radiograph. It may be so difficult to assess the degree of displacement of a lateral condylar fragment on plain films that arthrographic studies are necessary.

Displaced fractures of the lateral condyle often show a marked rotation of the fragment because of pull on it by the lateral ligamentous system and the forearm extensor mass. This is not amenable to closed reduction; therefore, operative treatment is required. It is apparent that whatever the form of the lateral condylar fracture, experienced orthopaedic advice is warranted.

Avulsion of the Medial Epicondyle

The medial epicondyle is an apophysis that may be avulsed by vigorous traction exerted by the medial ligamentous system or the forearm flexor mass. When it is significantly displaced, the medial epicondylar fracture requires open reduction and internal fixation. Medial epicondyles begin to ossify in children at about age 5 and, therefore, are not visible on plain radiographs prior to that time. Hence, when a child younger than age 5 has an elbow injury with major findings on the medial aspect but a radiograph that appears normal, one needs to consider a displaced medial epicondyle. Orthopaedic consultation with a view to manipulation under anesthesia may be necessary to clarify the diagnosis, although more sophisticated radiographic modalities, if available, may demonstrate the as yet uncalcified epicondyle.

Elbow Dislocation

Dislocated elbows are rare in children because of the relative weakness of bone or epiphyseal plate when compared with that of ligaments. A child tends to break the end of a bone before he or she dislocates the adjacent joint, and this is as true with the elbow as it is with any other joint.

The diagnosis of elbow dislocation can usually be made on clinical grounds. Generally there is clearly visible posterior displacement of the olecranon behind the elbow without the diffuse marked soft tissue edema of a supracondylar fracture. The lateral radiograph will show the humerus sitting in front of the coronoid process. Reduction is usually easy but should be confirmed by radiograph.

To permit dislocation, a tear or at least stretch of one or other of the collateral ligaments is necessary. However, in the child the medial epicondyle will pull off before the ligament ruptures. This explains the common association of elbow dislocation and avulsion of the medial epicondyle. When a dislocated elbow is treated, careful attention must be directed to the position of the medial epicondyle. Conversely, when a medial epicondylar avulsion is encountered, one cannot help but wonder if an elbow dislocation had been present, if only for a moment. When the child under age 5 presents with a dislocated elbow, particular concern regarding the medial epicondyle is warranted because the plain films will be of no help in locating the as yet uncalcified medial epicondyle.

Pulled Elbow (Nursemaid's Elbow)

"Pulled elbow" is a common lesion of the elbow in children from 1 to 4 years old. It is also seen infrequently in children up to 6 years old and occasionally in the first year of life.

The typical history is that of a sudden pull on the hand caused when a child walking hand-in-hand with a parent falls or is lifted up over a curb. An older child may inflict a pulled elbow by swinging a toddler about by the arms. The pulled elbow can sometimes be produced when a child slips from a climbing apparatus while holding on to it with one arm. When this condition is produced, there will be immediate pain and unwillingness to use the arm.

There are several theories for the pathology of the pulled elbow. Most experts believe that the longitudinal pull tears the thin, weak reflection of the annular ligament onto the radial neck. This is thought to remove the distal tether of the annular ligament and permits it to slip proximally into the radiocapitellar joint, causing pain and limiting supination.

In understanding the reduction maneuver, one should realize that the radial head itself, when visualized end-on, is oval and not truly circular. It is assumed that supination brings its longer axis into the anteroposterior direction, thus forcing the misplaced ligament out of the joint.

On examination the arm typically hangs dependent and pronated or alternatively is supported by the opposite arm with the elbow somewhat flexed. Although the child is not usually in much discomfort at this stage, he or she will refuse to use the arm, which gives the appearance of being paralyzed. Careful palpation, from clavicle to hand, will usually convince the examiner that there is little if any of the tenderness one would expect with a fracture. With the child distracted, a fair range of flexion and extension can usually be demonstrated, although the extremes will be resisted.

The examiner should then grasp the child's hand with one hand and support the elbow with the other. With the elbow held at about 90 degrees, the forearm should be briskly and firmly twisted into full supination. There will be resistance to supination and discomfort produced by it. The physician can be confident that the displaced ligament has reduced when this maneuver causes a palpable and often audible "clunk" perceived over the radial head and the child begins to use the elbow normally at once or in a very few minutes. If there has been no palpable clunk, one may wait for a few minutes before repeating the maneuver because the reduction is not always easily felt. A pulled elbow that remains out after one attempted reduction deserves one more concerted effort to reduce it. If supination does not result in a clunk, the physician should retain his or her grip on the arm and then firmly twist it into full pronation. Sometimes pronation succeeds when supination has failed.

One will occasionally encounter a child whose pulled elbow resists all attempts at reduction. A day in a sling may be tried because the child sometimes reduces the pulled elbow during that time. If so, the child will suddenly begin to use the arm at home and need not return. The pulled elbow that resists reduction can be expected to correct itself at home during the next few days.

An unusual variant of the typical pulled elbow occurs from time to time in the first year of life. The posture of the arm is typical for pulled elbow, but there may be no clear history of a pull. It is thought that a pull somehow has been exerted on the arm when it became trapped under the baby's body as he or she was rolled over by an older child or adult. Manipulative reduction has been as successful with the small baby as with the toddler.

Recurrent pulled elbows are seen from time to time; there is no evidence that there is any predisposing anatomic variation in such instances. One must be assured that the parents understand what produces a pulled elbow and that longitudinal pulls on the forearm should be avoided. Once successfully reduced, there does not seem to be any untoward sequelae from pulled elbows, even in those children who have had a number of episodes.

If the diagnosis is fairly convincing and there is no marked tenderness to suggest a fracture, there is no need for radiographic evaluation. Radiographs are warranted only in atypical situations, such as when the history is unclear, there is persistent failure to reduce, or there is significant tenderness.

Fracture-Separation of the Proximal Radial Epiphysis

The type II fracture of the proximal radial epiphysis is the pediatric analog of the radial head fracture in the adult. It is usually only minimally displaced and necessitates 3 weeks in a sling, or a cast if there is marked discomfort, with a perfect outcome to be expected. When there is significant angulation, reduction may be necessary. Closed manipulation with direct pressure over the head is usually sufficient; however, the occasional case requires open operation.

Forearm Fractures

Fractures of the shafts of the radius, ulna, or both are common. Displaced fractures of mid-shaft or distal shaft usually necessitate general or regional anesthesia to permit satisfactory reduction. In the mature child, however, the slightly angulated fracture which can be reduced with one quick maneuver may sometimes be efficiently handled under local infiltration or intravenous analgesia. Plaster immobilization for 6 weeks is indicated in most cases. Displaced fractures of both radius and ulna can be handled with closed reduction almost without exception. This is in contrast to adult forearm fractures, most of which are treated operatively. If angulation and rotation have been dealt with, displacement is of relative concern only and the surgeon may choose to accept bayonet apposition in a particularly difficult case, especially in the younger child.

Bowing Fracture

From time to time one sees a radiograph following trauma in which one of the forearm bones displays a smooth curve clearly different from a comparison film of the opposite member. This is called a bowing fracture and is the net effect of a myriad of microfractures. Attempts to straighten out such fractured bones are difficult and often not very successful. Orthopaedic judgment and assistance are necessary in dealing with bowing fractures.

Monteggia Fracture-Dislocation

Occasionally a child is encountered who has an angulated fracture of the shaft of the ulna with an intact radius. The ulna is shortened, while the radius is of normal length. For the radius and ulna to retain their normal relationship distally, it is clear that the radius must move proximally. This can occur only if the radial head has dislocated and is no longer stopped from moving proximally by the capitellum, with which it normally articulates. This is the Monteggia fracture-dislocation. Because in most such injuries the force has been applied to the dorsum of the arm, the radial head dislocates anteriorly and the ulnar fracture angulates anteriorly. This is the anterior Monteggia fracture-dislocation. Posterior Monteggia lesions are rare.

Sometimes a radiocapitellar dislocation is associated with a bowing fracture of the ulna. Hence, when this type of ulnar fracture is encountered, the Monteggia combination of lesions must be sought in the same way as it is with a displaced ulnar shaft fracture.

It is important for all primary contact physicians to be well acquainted with the Monteggia fracture-dislocation. Although the ulnar fracture is not easily missed, it may direct attention away from the associated dislocation, leading to the radial head being left in the dislocated position. This has important long-term sequelae even if the dislocation is subsequently recognized and treated.

The principle to be remembered with these injuries is as follows: *whenever there is an angulated ulnar shaft fracture with an intact radius, one must look for a radiocapitellar dislocation.* When one looks for a dislocated radial head on the radiograph, it is useful to remember that a straight line drawn up the center of the proximal radius should bisect the capitellum when extended across the joint. This applies regardless of the radiographic projection and regardless of the position of the elbow.

Another much less common combination injury is the Galeazzi fracture-dislocation. In this lesion, there is an angulated radial shaft fracture in addition to disruption of the distal radioulnar ligaments and proximal displacement of the distal end of the radius.

Greenstick Fractures

Shaft fractures in which the bone breaks through the convex portion of the shaft but bends in the concave part, akin to a partially broken green stick, are fairly common. When the angulation is enough to require reduction, the surgeon will need to overcorrect the angulation, in effect completing the fracture, to prevent recurrence of the original angulation. To ensure maintenance of the position that has been achieved, careful molding of the cast is essential.

Buckle Fractures
(Torus Fractures)

A buckle fracture can be considered to be a variant of a greenstick fracture in which the convex aspect of the bone bends and the concave portion breaks. The difference between a buckle fracture and the usual greenstick fracture is that the fracture component demonstrates crumpling inward on itself of the bony architecture, not breaking apart as is the case with a greenstick fracture. Buckle fractures are very common near the ends of long bones, particularly the radius.

When a child falls on the hand and arrives in the emergency department with an "injured wrist," the location of the tenderness must be identified. When tenderness is over the dorsum of the distal radius, the likely diagnosis is a buckle fracture of the radius, even if the fracture is not easily seen on the radiograph. Many children who are shown to have buckle fractures seek help only after 3 or 4 days because soreness has persisted. Others go through the whole course of healing without seeking medical assistance because function may not be greatly restricted. Most buckle fractures would heal uneventfully if untreated because they are quite stable. However, in the majority of instances there is sufficient tenderness to warrant plaster protection for 3 weeks. This eliminates the pain that ensues when the child rolls over in bed, striking the arm on a firm object, and provides for almost normal activity immediately after cast removal.

The buckle which shows appreciable compression fracturing of the dorsal cortex or in which there is marked pain on pronation or supination may not be totally stable. It should be immobilized in a cast extending from metacarpal heads to the axilla that is carefully molded into pronation to prevent the further angulation that might result were supination permitted.

Wringer Injuries

Although the majority of clothes wringers have been replaced by spin driers, there are still a few wringers in use or available as second-hand items, and wringer injuries are still seen, albeit infrequently. Industrial wringer injuries caused by large roller presses occur from time to time but are rarely, if ever, seen in the pediatric institution.

The wringer injury seen in pediatric practice characteristically occurs in the 3- to 7-year-old child, who, through curiosity and lack of understanding of the potential danger, has permitted the hand to enter the gap between the moving rollers of a wringer. Once the hand has been pulled in even a short distance it is virtually impossible to extract it without releasing the rollers. In many wringer injuries, the arm is drawn in until it is finally stopped at the axilla, where the rollers continue to churn over the same tissue. Sometimes the older child or adult who arrives on the scene then reverses the rollers and the arm is traumatized again as it is extruded. On other occasions, whoever attempts the rescue manages to free the arm by literally pulling it out against the pull of the rollers, thus adding greatly to the friction forces. Although most wringers have a release control that allows the rollers to separate immediately, this is often ignored in the heat of the moment.

The mechanical forces that cause the damage are a combination of friction, grinding, shearing, and direct compression. These forces burn skin and contuse muscle, nerve, and blood vessel. Skin can be sheared away from underlying layers and consequently from its vascular supply. Hematomas lifting skin away from deeper layers can also be instrumental in rendering it ischemic. Major muscle contusion can result in enough muscle edema to cause a compartment syndrome with additional muscle damage from hypoxia. Fractures are rare complications of wringer injuries.

Although in the extreme wringer injuries can be of calamitous proportions, fortunately these are rare. Most injuries involve no more than the hand or the hand and lower forearm. Minor abrasions and contusions are usually the extent of the damage. In these cases, little treatment and brief follow-up are usually adequate. Nevertheless, the initial appearance of the injury rarely indicates the true severity of the underlying damage, and more serious pathology must be suspected. Because of this, frequent follow-up examinations must be insisted on, particularly if the child is to be treated as an outpatient.

Radiographs are requested for the majority of wringer injuries, although fractures are unusual.

Superficial burns or scrapes should be cleansed and dressed appropriately. Most physicians now believe that a compression bandage does not improve outcome and may act only to limit surveillance of the area. Immunization against tetanus must be confirmed. For even minor wringer injuries, elevation of the arm for the first 24 to 48 hours is important. Finally, the crucial element in management is frequent examination for assessment of soft tissue viability. This permits increasing pressure from edema or hematoma formation to be detected and decompressed on an emergency basis.

In the very rare situation of a serious wringer injury, admission to the hospital and close observation is warranted.

Wrist Fractures

Carpal scaphoid fractures are unusual in children under the age of 13 or 14 but begin to be encountered after that age in increasing frequency. Their management is similar to the treatment applied in the adult age group. Other fractures or fracture dislocations of the wrist bones are rare in the pediatric age group.

Sprains of the Wrist

Before the diagnosis of wrist sprain should ever be accepted, concerted effort must be made to rule out a buckle fracture of the distal radius, fracture-separation of the distal radial epiphysis, or the much less common scaphoid fracture. Sprains are very uncommon because of the strength of the ligaments when compared with the bones or epiphyses. The forces that would result in a sprain in an adult can be expected to cause a fracture in the child.

Fractures of the Hand

Injuries to the proximal ends of the metacarpals are uncommon and usually undisplaced when they occur. However, a type II fracture-separation of the epiphysis of the first metacarpal is seen from time to time and is the pediatric analog of Bennett's fracture in the adult. Reduction is not often required.

Metacarpal shaft fractures are common. However, unless several bones are broken, displacement is usually minimal and reduction is rarely needed.

Fractures of the distal ends of the metacarpals are also common; they may be epiphyseal separations or may be situated proximal to the plate. The most common such fracture occurs at the end of the fifth metacarpal as the result of a blow by the closed fist on a wall or doorjamb. In these, the knuckle usually looks depressed, and on the radiograph volar displacement of the head is customary. Reduction is difficult, and unless the deformity is marked and has occurred in an older child with little remolding potential, it is seldom worthwhile to attempt it.

Phalangeal fractures may be of many varieties. Epiphyseal fracture-separations are common, particularly involving the proximal phalanx of the fifth finger, which may display abduction deformity at the fracture site to the extent that reduction is warranted. Reduction can usually be accomplished simply with regional or local infiltration anesthesia. Mid-shaft fractures may also demonstrate sufficient angulation, both on clinical examination and on radiograph, that reduction is necessary. Terminal phalangeal tuft fractures are common components of fingertip compression injuries so often produced in younger children who have gotten fingers caught in doors, drawers, or windows. However, the associated injury to the nail bed and touch pad is more important, and the tuft fracture can usually be ignored.

Plaster cast protection of metacarpal fractures is frequently warranted, if only from the point of view of comfort. Plaster or other forms of splints may also serve the purpose very well. For most finger fractures, padded aluminum splints can be cut and formed to shape and should maintain the position satisfactorily for the week or two required. Finger fractures and epiphyseal fractures in the hand are generally united within 1½ to 2 weeks, whereas metacarpal fractures may require immobilization for 2 to 3 weeks depending on the age of the child.

After epiphyseal closure, avulsion of the ventral-proximal corner of the middle phalanx is common and probably represents an avulsion of the bony attachment of the palmar plate along with the insertion of the flexor digitorum superficialis.

The majority of these fractures can be handled by simple splintage; however, some show significant deformity, and surgical advice should be sought if there is any question. Similarly fractures representing avulsions of tendinous insertions warrant consultation because some of these will need internal fixation after reduction.

Subungual Hematoma

The pediatric fingertip is frequently caught and squeezed in doors, drawers, or closing windows or is unexpectedly compressed between a rock and the ground or between somebody's heel and the floor. Trauma of this nature frequently results in an accumulation of blood under the nail. The cause is usually a small, transversely directed laceration of the nail bed. It should be recognized that bone lies exposed in the depths of this laceration, and if there is communication to the outside through or around the nail, there is potential contamination of bone.

Some subungual hematomas are small, obviously not under much pressure, and do not cause much discomfort. These require no treatment. Other hematomas are under significant pressure, as is evidenced by the considerable throbbing pain. When the child cannot sleep because of the discomfort and walks into the department holding the hand up in the air there is clearly enough pain to warrant release of the blood.

Decompression of a subungual hematoma can be accomplished in a number of ways. A convenient, battery-powered, rechargeable electrocautery tool has been designed for this procedure that burns through the nail easily and painlessly. The old-fashioned red-hot paper clip works, but is it difficult to keep the metal from plunging into the tender nail bed when it suddenly penetrates the nail. If there is access to dental equipment, an easy method is to drill the nail with a dental bur. Whatever method is selected, the pain is dramatically relieved as soon as the subungual space has been entered.

The only significant complication to this procedure is subungual infection in the remnants of the clot. To avoid this, the hole must be large enough to permit adequate drainage, and efforts must be made to express as much of the blood as possible by pressing on the nail all around the hole. One may then attempt to minimize the risk of reaccumulation of blood by the application of a tight bandage for a short period of time.

Large subungual hematomas, in which the nail appears to be floating on a "lake" of blood, are usually under little pressure and not particularly painful. However, rather than wait until the nail detaches itself and the blood escapes, nail removal and cleansing of the area under aseptic conditions are preferable. When the entire nail is elevated by the clot, it can often be removed without anesthesia by dividing the elevated cuticular tissue around the margins of the nail. Although the laceration in the nail bed will then be evident, it is usually not amenable to repair. Dressing under asepsis is indicated.

Fingertip Injuries

The small subungual hematoma should probably be considered the least severe form of fingertip injury. Various grades of damage to the tip occur with more violent forces. Generally, however, the injury appears as if the tip has been pulled distally and ventrally, with the lacerations usually on the dorsal surface and the remaining attachment to the finger on the ventral surface.

An initial stage occurs when the nail is pulled out of its proximal nail fold and is seen to be riding external to the eponychia. A further stage displays the nail pulled out still more with a laceration across the nail bed. Deepening of the laceration across the nail bed, with extension down each side, results in a partial amputation, with the tip suspended on a ventral flap revealing the bony tuft of the terminal phalanx. In most instances, regardless of extent of the tissue avulsion, the nail usually remains attached to the distal part of the nail bed.

Radiographs usually reveal a fracture of the phalangeal tuft, and it may even be visible when the finger is examined carefully. Specific treatment for this fracture is rarely warranted.

Surgical repair of this lesion, regardless of the severity, is usually accomplished easily under digital block anesthesia, provided that the tip remains viable. Skin sutures on either side of the nail usually hold the tip in place accurately, and it is sometimes feasible to place one or two absorbable sutures in the nail bed itself.

More efforts are being put lately into replacement of the avulsed nail into the nail fold beneath the eponychia in an attempt to prevent subsequent adherence of the cleft and to provide a splint for the nail bed itself in the event of damage to it at the time of the injury. This remains somewhat speculative because a great many nails have been removed over the years for one reason or another without any resulting abnormality of the regenerating nail. However, if replacement of the nail can be done easily, any added measure to help ensure normal nail regeneration is warranted.

When surgical repair is required, fingertip injuries are best handled under tourniquet-induced ischemia. A narrow Penrose drain pulled tightly and held in place by a surgical clamp around the proximal segment of the finger is an effective tourniquet. The repair should be completed, a snug bandage applied, and the hand elevated before the tourniquet is removed. The outcome of these repairs is usually very good, provided that the avulsed tip was completely viable.

Splinters

Splinters under a fingernail are common occurrences and should be removed to prevent infection. The methods of achieving anesthesia and removal of splinters are discussed in Chapter 9.

Lower Extremity Injuries

Apophyseal Avulsions Around the Hip

The lesser trochanter, the ischial tuberosity, the anterior inferior iliac spine, and the anterior superior iliac spine are occasionally avulsed by sudden violent contraction of the iliopsoas muscle, the hamstrings, the rectus femoris muscle, and the sartorius muscle, respectively. These lesions are typically seen in the adolescent sprinter or skater who has attempted to take a vigorous stride forward.

Most such avulsions reveal a separation of only a very few millimeters, and satisfactory union is usually achieved without surgical intervention. Symptomatic treatment and avoidance of vigorous activity for several weeks suffice in most instances. These separations cross sites of active endochondral ossification and heal faster than would the pulled or torn tendon, the analogous injury in the adult.

Slipped Femoral Capital Epiphysis

Displacement of the femoral capital epiphysis can be considered the pediatric analog of the transcervical fracture of the elderly. The femoral head epiphysis can be knocked right off the femoral shaft by a single violent traumatic episode, causing a clinical picture similar to an adult with a displaced transcervical fracture, with shortening and external rotation. However, the usual story is one of mild to moderate pain, with limp, going on for weeks before investigation reveals an early or partial slip or before further mechanical stress then results in the head slipping right off.

Pain and limp are the classic symptoms in the early stages and usually occur within the 2 or 3 years prior to closure of the femoral capital epiphysis (i.e., age 10 to 14 in the girl and 12 to 16 in the boy). The pain is most commonly situated in the groin and initially occurs only during vigorous activity but gradually comes to be noted with almost any activity. The pain may also be noted in the thigh or knee. Knee pain in a young teenager who seems to have a normal knee on examination should alert one to the possible presence of hip disease.

Examination may be singularly unrewarding, unless there has been a recent significant slip of the head resulting in pain with movement. One may note a tendency for the hip to roll into slight external rotation as it is passively flexed. When the femoral head has slipped appreciably, there may be limitation of flexion.

Unfortunately some children with early and slight epiphyseal slips may be totally free of pain when seen and may have no or minimal physical findings. The majority, however, will show a tendency toward slight external rotation on walking and often a very slight Trendelenburg gait.

The physician must be alert to the slipped capital epiphysis as almost the only serious disease that can appear in this manner in an otherwise completely well child. One must rule out this condition in such children because the consequences of permitting a partially slipped femoral head to slip off completely can be disastrous. Even though the orthopaedic surgeon reduces the totally displaced head accurately and pins it there, there is still a 25 to 35 percent risk of it undergoing infarction, which despite satisfactory short-term results is likely to cause a crippling osteoarthritis within 10 to 15 years. Conversely, with slight or partial slips, pinning in situ almost invariably produces excellent results.

Whenever a slipped femoral capital epiphysis is a possibility, radiographs of the upper femur are necessary. Because the femoral epiphysis tends to slip posteriorly, the displacement is best seen and sometimes only seen on the lateral projection. In pediatric practice, the simplest and most convenient way to obtain a lateral view of the upper femur is by use of the froglike position, in which the hips and knees are flexed and the hips then externally rotated until the knees are as close to the bed on either side as is possible without the use of undue force. An anteroposterior view taken with the child in the froglike position gives an anteroposterior view of the acetabula but a lateral view of the upper femora.

When radiographs are requested because a slipped femoral epiphysis is suspected, weight bearing must be avoided until the radiographs are interpreted as normal. It is disastrous when hip pain is noted and an epiphyseal slip is considered, but investigation is delayed until "we see if it will get better," only to have the femoral head displaced further in the interim.

Fractures of the Hip

Hip fractures are rare in children and require a great deal of force before they occur, in contrast to the often trivial force that may result in a fractured hip in an older person. Direct longitudinal force up the long axis of the femur may produce a transcervical fracture. This may be seen in the child who strikes the knee against the dashboard on being thrown forward in a head-on collision. Torsion is more likely to produce a subtrochanteric or intertrochanteric fracture. The clinical presentation of a fractured hip in a child is similar to that described in adults, with external rotation and shortening.

The treatment of the transcervical fracture in a child is also similar to that in adults. However, the magnitude of mechanical force required to produce a transcervical fracture is greater in children, and the more severe trauma that this implies also means that the risk of avascular necrosis of the femoral head is greater. Hence, the overall prognosis is worse. Hip fractures below the cervical level can be expected to unite strongly and rapidly and are treated either in traction if in reasonably good position or with internal fixation. All hip fractures in children must be considered as serious injuries that are prone to complications and in need of experienced orthopaedic care.

Hip Dislocation

Dislocations of the hip are distinctly uncommon in children. Such dislocations usually require general anesthesia for reduction. Sophisticated orthopaedic attention is also necessary.

Posterior dislocations occur when, with a flexed hip, the femoral shaft is driven backward. There is often an acetabular fracture as well. These fractures present with the hip in fixed adduction and flexion and show apparent shortening of the thigh.

Anterior dislocations occur when the thigh has been forced into excessive abduction and may be seen when a child on a toboggan or sled comes too close to a tree, which then forces the child's knee violently out to the side and back. When a child seems to have the hip stuck out in wide abduction, an anterior dislocation is a strong possibility.

The dislocation may be evident on an anteroposterior view alone. However, one cannot rule out dislocation with one apparently normal view. A cross-table lateral view may be necessary to reveal the displacement of the head in the anteroposterior plane.

The longer the head is out of the hip joint, the greater is the incidence of avascular necrosis. Because of this, there must be no delay in referring the patient for reduction of the dislocation.

Proximal Femoral Shaft Fractures

Fractures of the proximal shaft display the same tendency for the proximal fragment to flex at the hip as is seen in the older patient. The need to immobilize with the distal shaft aligned with the proximal fragment is apparent. In children, this is usually achieved by applying

90 degree–90 degree traction, with both hip and knee flexed to a right angle and the femur controlled by a distal pin inserted in such a way as to avoid the growth plate.

Mid-Shaft Femoral Fractures

Fractures of the shaft are common in children, both as isolated injuries, often caused by torsional stress, or as components in the multiple injury complex caused by pedestrian-vehicle accidents.

Unlike the outcome of this lesion in adults, it is unusual for a femoral shaft fracture in a child to cause enough interstitial hemorrhage to produce the clinical picture of hypovolemic shock. When a child with a fractured femur demonstrates the tachycardia and hypotension of hemorrhagic shock, he or she is probably bleeding from a ruptured spleen, liver, or kidney or has a hemopneumothorax.

The femoral shaft fracture is usually diagnosed by the prehospital care attendant who first reaches the child or by the nurse who receives the child in the emergency department. Swelling and deformity of the mid-thigh, apparent shortening, and severe pain on any movement all point to a fractured femur.

Careful general assessment of the patient is necessary so as not to miss associated injuries. If there is any doubt concerning the presence of other injuries, blood should be obtained for crossmatching and a venous infusion established. However, this is not likely to be needed if the femoral fracture is the only significant injury.

The initial care for most femoral fractures is also the definitive treatment. Longitudinal skin traction in a Thomas splint restores alignment in most instances and should be applied before any radiographs are obtained. This measure stabilizes the bony fragments while the patient is subsequently moved, undergoes radiographic examination, and is transferred to the ward. Any radiograph of an unstable femoral shaft fracture in its early stages that does not also demonstrate the presence of the splint implies inferior care. To avoid undue longitudinal tension on the femoropopliteal arterial tree while in the splint, the knee should be flexed a few degrees. This is accomplished by simply bending the Thomas splint a few degrees in the appropriate direction at the level of the knee.

During the manipulation, which is part of the process of application of the traction, analgesia is in order. However, care must be taken to ensure that there are no associated injuries the symptoms of which might be masked by the analgesic drug.

Subsequent to the application of the traction, radiographs will confirm the diagnosis and permit adjustment of the traction if this is necessary. Admission will be required for approximately 3 to 4 weeks, depending on the age of the child. This period in traction maintains length and alignment until the fracture is sufficiently "sticky" that protection in a cast is sufficient. The traction is then removed and replaced by a plaster hip spica in which the child goes home. A rough estimate of the number of weeks of immobilization that will be required, including time both in traction and in cast, can be obtained by adding four to the child's age in years.

Operative repair of a femoral shaft fracture is rarely indicated in the young child. One exception is the child who is very restless and thrashing about because of an associated head injury. In these children, intramedullary nailing removes the need for the traction apparatus and greatly facilitates nursing care. On the other hand, there is an increasing tendency toward internal fixation in children over 12 years of age.

Over the years, femoral shaft fractures have been more prone than most fractures to Volkmann's ischemic contracture, as a result of direct vascular injury sustained at the initial trauma, secondary vascular spasm, or a combination of the two. For this reason, careful observation for the symptoms and signs of ischemia is essential during the first few days in traction. Pain in the calf muscle bulk due to hypoxic cellular swelling within the closed fascial compartment is the usual early symptom of ischemia and is made much worse by passive stretch or by active contraction of the muscles involved. It should be emphasized that muscular pain can be due to ischemia even in the presence of a palpable dorsalis pedis pulse. When a femoral shaft fracture has been immobilized in traction, pain is usually well controlled, so persistent pain, especially in the calf, must be assumed to be of ischemic origin.

It has been shown that longitudinal stretch is the form of mechanical stress which, more than most others, causes spasm of an arterial tree. Therefore, when calf pain and tenderness, or any other evidence of muscle ischemia, occur, immediate removal of the traction force is necessary to eliminate longitudinal stretch from the vascular tree. For this reason, immediate repositioning of the patient into the horizontal plane and slight flexion of the knee are first steps. If the symptoms subside rapidly, attention may be redirected to the fracture, which will need to be treated in a manner that does not again stretch the femoropopliteal system. If this initial maneuver does not induce clear improvement in the symptoms and signs, immediate attention to the state of the vascular tree is required. This will probably entail arteriography and exploration and cannot be delayed lest permanent loss of muscle function be the result.

The niceties of the application of the traction apparatus, the decisions as to the acceptable bony position from day to day, the judgments required to decide when discharge in plaster is safe, and the risk of vascular complications while in traction are all sophisticated orthopaedic considerations. For this reason, fractured femurs should be under the care of a surgical consultant.

Distal Femoral Fractures

When there is a fracture near the lower end of the femur, posterior angulation may be produced by the gastrocnemius muscle as it tries to "flex" the knee. In this situation, more flexion of the knee in the traction is necessary to align the bony fragments.

Type II fracture-separation of the lower femoral epiphysis can usually be reduced with little difficulty and the position maintained in either plaster or traction. On examination, this lesion can be mistaken for a medial ligamentous disruption because pronounced valgus deformity may be apparent. When this is the case, stress views may be necessary to demonstrate the fracture. On occasion one condyle may be knocked off, producing a type III or IV epiphyseal injury. These usually require operative reduction and fixation.

Toddler's Femoral Fracture

Undisplaced buckle fractures, usually of the distal shaft, or stable hairline cracks in the mid-shaft area, often requiring several views for adequate visualization, are seen from time to time in the toddler age group, although they are not nearly as common as the toddler fracture of the tibia. Unstable fractures in this age group require the customary form of treatment, with traction followed by plaster immobilization. However, many fractures are completely stable and do not require definitive treatment unless pain warrants it. Many can be treated without plaster, with a month or so of no weight bearing. Although femoral fractures at all levels are common accidental injuries of childhood, abuse should be kept in mind, particularly in the child under 2 years of age and especially for mid-shaft fractures.

Disruptions of Knee Ligaments

The ligamentous injuries that are occasionally seen in children tend to be in older teenagers because the ligaments of younger children are more resistant to stretch than are the epiphyseal plates to disruption. For this reason, whenever a child is seen with an injured knee which in an adult would suggest a torn ligament, care must be taken to look for an epiphyseal injury to either the distal femur or the proximal tibia. With a clearly unstable knee, examination under anesthesia with the help of stress radiographs may be necessary to identify the site of the instability.

Recurrent Dislocation of the Patella

Kneecap dislocation is a common lesion in children between the ages of 14 and 18. Predisposing factors are (1) knock-knees or genu valgus, (2) a flattened lateral femoral condyle, and (3) weak quadriceps muscles, particularly the vastus medialis. In such an individual, the valgus deformity of the knee results in the patella being pulled laterally when the quadriceps muscles contract. Once a dislocation has occurred, the medial restraining tissues, particularly the insertion of the vastus medialis, are stretched and fail in tethering the patella medially. As a result, subsequent dislocations occur more readily and often with trivial force. The usual history is that the episode occurred when the subject was undergoing a twisting motion, such as when hitting a baseball.

Genu valgus is seen more frequently in girls than in boys. Similarly recurrent patellar dislocation is more frequent in girls.

Visualization of the kneecap displaced well lateral to its normal site makes the diagnosis easy. Reduction is usually easy also. The knee should be gradually extended fully. This is moderately painful and may require analgesia, unless it has happened several times before. If the patella does not reduce spontaneously with extension, it is an easy matter to push it back to the front of the knee once extension has been achieved. When one individual has had several previous episodes, not only does dislocation seem to be more readily produced, but also reduction is easier and less painful.

If the dislocation has been a momentary episode followed by spontaneous reduction, the diagnosis is much more difficult. The history of a twisting motion as the precipitating incident is suggestive. There will probably be some blood in the joint, although this is variable. Tenderness medially and just above the joint level is also suggestive because it may indicate a tear in the insertion of the vastus medialis. The patellar apprehension test may be useful. In this test, pushing the patella laterally should induce a protective contraction of the quadriceps if a recent episode of dislocation has occurred. If there is no protective quadriceps contraction, a recent patellar dislocation is highly unlikely.

After reduction, a bulky pressure bandage will provide adequate temporary splintage. Elective orthopaedic consultation is indicated to obtain follow-up advice and to permit any necessary decisions regarding surgical correction. There are several successful operative procedures available to prevent recurrences, and after several episodes consideration must be given to more definitive therapy.

Fractures Within the Knee

In osteochondritis dissecans, a small osteochondral fragment usually separates from the medial surface of the lateral femoral condyle. There is generally no single episode of trauma to which the "fracture" can be attributed, and some form of local degeneration must be considered in the etiology. The fragment behaves as a "joint mouse" and can give the picture of a torn meniscus. The radiograph may show nothing of note, although in many instances one can see a small bony fragment within the joint and even the defect in the femoral condyle where it originated. The fragment is largely cartilage, and unless the bony part of it is large enough to be seen on radiograph, the diagnosis remains presumptive. Previous episodes of locking would be supportive of the diagnosis. Orthopaedic advice is needed to decide on further investigation and definitive care.

Fracture of the tibial spine, although uncommon, does occur and is the pediatric analog of a torn anterior cruciate ligament. In the child, the strong ligament remains intact and pulls the tibial spine out of the upper tibial surface. This will produce a distended, blood-filled knee. There will be pain and abnormally free forward tibial mobility on testing for the anterior cruciate ligament. The fragment is rarely more than slightly displaced and will usually reduce satisfactorily in extension. Future stability of the knee is at stake with this injury, and careful orthopaedic consideration is necessary.

Patellar Fracture

Broken kneecaps are uncommon in pediatric practice. A congenital bipartite patella is seen from time to time and can be readily confused with a fracture. Unless there is marked tenderness over the site, fracture need not be seriously considered. Congenital bipartite patellae are usually bilateral, and radiograph of the opposite knee may clarify the issue if there is concern regarding radiographic interpretation.

Fractures of the Tibial Shaft

Tibial shaft fractures, with or without fracture of the fibula, are caused by vehicular accidents, falls from a height, or sports injuries. The possibility of abuse must be kept in mind, although tibial fractures are not often due to abuse.

As in adults, some tibial shaft fractures are open and require appropriately aggressive surgical care.

Occasionally one sees a transverse fracture close to the upper end of the tibia, which tends to open up on the medial side, readily permitting a valgus deformity at the level of the fracture. Immobilization in a cast with the knee extended and molded into varus may be necessary to prevent this valgus tendency during the first several weeks in plaster.

The "toddler's tibial fracture" is common in the child from about 1 year of age to 3 or 4. It may be an almost indiscernible buckle of the lower tibial cortex, or it may be a barely visible oblique hairline crack crossing the lower third. The child is likely to have fallen a relatively short distance, in which case nothing significant is suspected until the crying is noted to persist for 20 or 30 minutes. It is then observed that the child holds the foot off the floor when lifted into the standing position. Although most such children will refuse to bear weight and may revert to crawling, some are still able to walk and may even limp into the department, bearing weight on the leg.

Tenderness over the tibia is the clue to the diagnosis; however, the child's persistent crying may make it difficult to locate the site of the tenderness. When the child cries through the whole examination, one may be tempted to take the easy way out and obtain radiographs of the entire leg from hip to toes. Not only is this unnecessary, but also it is unwarranted radiation and indicates in most instances that the physician did not take the time required to examine the child properly.

Locating the site of extremity tenderness in a crying child can be difficult and is often time-consuming. With such children, withdrawal of the limb is the chief response to be watched for. First one should gently but firmly palpate the good leg, gradually moving up from toes to thigh, until the child is accustomed to feeling hands on the leg. One then switches surreptitiously to the other leg, again starting at the distal part of the foot and working up, all the while attempting to distract the child's attention from the palpating hand. Care must be taken to apply firm but gentle pressure only, without indirect stress or moving any joint. When the leg is suddenly pulled away, a point of tenderness has been reached. This whole process should be repeated several times. Repeated withdrawal with palpation at the same site identifies the point of tenderness. A radiograph will probably reveal an undisplaced fracture.

When the standard radiographic projections seem normal, oblique projections may demonstrate the fracture. Some toddler's fractures do not show up on any films, and short of resorting to bone scan or computed tomography, radiographic proof of the diagnosis may have to await the development of periosteal new bone, visible by radiograph 8 to 10 days later.

With most tibial shaft fractures in toddlers, solid union is obtained with immobilization in plaster for 3 to 6 weeks, depending on the child's age, although the chief purpose of the cast is to relieve pain.

When the radiograph is equivocal and the history of trauma is not clear, the leg should not be hidden behind plaster until the clinical situation is clarified, lest early osteomyelitis be obscured by the cast. However, with localized tenderness over the lower third of a tibia following a clearly described traumatic episode, even when there is no radiographically demonstrated fracture, the presumptive diagnosis of shaft fracture is warranted. Although the fracture can be identified with a later radiograph, this may well be unjustified unless symptoms persist, since the child will be nearly recovered by then.

When a child is in pain and cannot sleep because of a toddler's fracture of the tibia, a long leg cast is warranted. On the other hand, such fractures can usually be expected to unite rapidly without plaster immobilization.

Fractures of the Distal Tibia

Fracture-separations of the lower tibial epiphysis are encountered frequently enough that the primary care physician needs to be aware of the variety which may be seen and of the prognosis attendant on each.

The type II separation of the distal tibial epiphysis occurs when the child is moving rapidly forward, as is the case when the child jumps forward only to have the foot suddenly stopped. This puts vigorous backward shearing force on the lower end of the tibia and is likely to displace the epiphysis in the posterior direction. The epiphysis almost always takes a posterior metaphyseal triangle of bone with it, becoming therefore a type II fracture. This posterior displacement may reduce spontaneously if the patient is placed in the prone position with the feet extending over the end of the stretcher. Others may require manipulation under general anesthesia to achieve satisfactory reduction. A long leg cast, carefully molded around the ankle, is the customary form of immobilization. Such a cast will be needed for 4 to 5 weeks, or roughly half as long as would be needed for a displaced tibial shaft fracture in a child of the same age. As is the outcome of most type II separations, there should be no growth disturbance unless the initial energy of impact had a vertical component strong enough to cause an additional type V lesion.

The Tillaux fracture, or type III separation of the lower tibial epiphysis, occurs in the 11- to 13-year-old girl or the 13- to 15-year-old boy. At this specific age, the state of partial closure of the epiphyseal plate predisposes to this lesion. The lower tibial epiphysis closes gradually from the medial side to the lateral and, hence, for a number of months is partially fused. Inversion and external rotation of the foot typically cause this lesion. When this occurs, the anterior tibiofibular ligaments pull the as yet unfused portion of the epiphysis laterally. There is usually minimal displacement, and plaster immobilization is generally sufficient treatment. However, when the gap in the articular surface of the tibia is greater than 2 mm, reduction should be considered. This can often be accomplished closed, but open operation is currently preferred by many orthopaedists. Growth would be a concern were this lesion seen in a younger child because the fracture does cross the growing cartilage zone. However, there is no growth left at this site to be affected by the Tillaux fracture.

One occasionally sees a type III fracture of the medial malleolus in a child whose epiphyses have not begun to fuse. In these cases, proper reduction is essential and is likely to require internal fixation to maintain.

A type IV fracture of the medial malleolar area may also be encountered and, similarly, requires perfect anatomic reduction to prevent cross union between the epiphysis and the metaphysis. This can result if there is any degree of upward displacement of the fragment. Internal fixation is required if the reduction is unstable to any degree.

In the triplanar fracture, the epiphyseal fracture line extends upward into the metaphysis at one site and down across the plate at another, producing a combination type II and III fracture. It is a difficult fracture to assess and treat and requires experienced orthopaedic care.

Type I Fracture-Separation, Lower Fibular Epiphysis

An inversion injury of the ankle in the child puts longitudinal stress on the lateral malleolus by pulling inferiorly on the talofibular ligament. When the force is great enough, this results in failure of the lateral collateral system at its weakest point, the epiphyseal plate, specifically at the zone of provisional calcification in the growth plate. This produces a type I epiphyseal fracture in contrast to the ligamentous tear, or ankle sprain, which would be the expected lesion in an adult.

The clinical presentation provides the diagnosis. When a clear history can be obtained, it will be that of an inversion injury. There will be swelling directly over the malleolus and not over the ligaments. Tenderness will be localized over the lateral malleolus and particularly over the plate itself.

The radiograph will show tissue swelling over the malleolus, but only very rarely will it show any bony abnormality. It is very unusual for the film to reveal any apparent widening of the epiphyseal plate, although occasionally there seems to be a crumb of bone off the metaphysis which suggests that some of these are actually type II injuries. This condition is diagnosed clinically in the vast majority of instances, and the purpose of the radiograph is chiefly to exclude other and less common bony injuries.

Epiphyseal separation of the lateral malleolus will heal solidly within 3 weeks, and if the degree of discomfort is mild, plaster immobilization is not always necessary, although crutches may be needed for a few days. If the soreness and pain are severe, a below-knee walking plaster worn for 3 weeks is appropriate. The activities of the child, where the child lives, and the severity of the clinical picture all play a part in the selection of treatment.

Lateral Malleolar Avulsions

In the younger teenager who still has unfused epiphyses, an inversion-adduction stress on the foot exerts a pull on the front of the tip of the malleolus by the anterior talofibular ligament. Rather than stretching or tearing the ligament, this is more likely to result in the avulsion of a small fragment of bone from the anterior surface of the lateral malleolus. Some physicians believe that pain and tenderness persisting over the site of this fragment for some weeks may be the outcome unless the ankle is carefully immobilized in a cast initially.

Sprained Ankle

In children an inversion stress to the ankle is more likely to produce a type I fracture-separation of the lower fibular epiphysis than a sprained ankle. However, sprained ankles are seen from time to time, especially in teenagers playing sports. Assessment of the severity of the injury and choice of treatment are similar to that in adult practice. Emphasis must be placed on early and active return to function except when severe disruption has occurred. Too often the mild sprain is aggravated by a regimen of tensor bandage and crutches, which does little more than increase the edema and stiffness unless combined with elevation and active exercise.

Bicycle Spoke Injury

The bicycle spoke injury is sustained characteristically by the small child who rides on the passenger seat mounted over the rear wheel of the parent's bicycle. Although newly manufactured seats of this nature have a protective shield over the upper half of the wheel, there are still many older seats that have no such guard. This permits the child's foot to become caught between two spokes and be carried forward by the rotating wheel until it is jammed tightly against the bicycle fork.

The injury sustained is produced by the compression and grinding forces exerted between spokes and fork. A severe contusion/abrasion is the result, with the trauma being sustained mainly by skin, subcutaneous tissue, and other soft tissues such as tendons and muscle. The visible lesion is usually localized to the area beneath and anterior to the lateral malleolus, although occasionally there is a comparable lesion medially. Fractures are described but are rare.

Basic care consists of appropriate dressing of any external wound, elevation, and observation. As is noted with wringer injuries, the ultimate damage is usually worse than is suggested by the initial appearance, and an important component of the care is continued surveillance until healing is complete. Unfortunately, of the skin contusion/abrasions that look innocuous initially, some will progress to local necrosis, ultimate sloughing, and ulceration. Occasionally skin grafting is required to repair the defect and cover underlying structures. Fortunately deeper damage of significance is uncommon.

Fractures of the Foot

Calcaneal fractures are unusual in children, although there have been recent suggestions that toddlers sustain calcaneal fractures more commonly than has been previously thought. Therefore, when an obscure leg injury has been sustained by a toddler, one should look particularly for both heel tenderness and tibial tenderness.

Metatarsal and toe fractures are common and rarely require more than symptomatic treatment. When there is doubt as to whether a line across the base of the fifth metatarsal represents a fracture or the apophysis, one should remember that a fracture almost always crosses the bone transversely. The apophysis is situated on the lateral side of the proximal end, and the plate is directed longitudinally.

Puncture Wounds of the Sole of the Foot

The nail puncture wound to the sole of the foot is a very common summertime injury, when outside activities in casual footwear or none at all is popular. These are caused by a wide variety of nails or similar objects, which possess a varying amount of visible soilage and invisible contamination. Questions when such a wound is encountered are as follows:

1. How deep did the nail go?
2. What was its direction?
3. Can the nail have penetrated to bone or joint?
4. Was the nail clean or dirty?
5. How long ago was the incident?
6. What footwear did the nail pierce?
7. Is a retained foreign body likely?
8. How much inflammation is already present?
9. What is the child's tetanus immunization status?

The location of the puncture wound on the sole of the foot is an important indicator of the likelihood of complications. Punctures over the metatarsal heads or more distally over the metatarsophalangeal joints or the toes are at particular risk of involving bone or joint. These structures are relatively close to the skin surface, and the majority of serious infections after nail puncture wounds are located distally. These infections usually involve bone or joint and are often due to *Pseudomonas aeruginosa*. Punctures over the heel are less likely to have penetrated to bone or result in major infection. If the perforation is in the mid area of the foot, the incidence of significant infection is even less.

Many nail punctures are so superficial and innocuous that medical help is not even sought. Not only do the majority of these punctures heal uneventfully, but also tetanus is very rarely seen because of the effectiveness of the general tetanus immunization program. Nevertheless, every nail puncture should be reviewed medically, if only to confirm proper tetanus immunization. There is great controversy regarding the care for nail puncture wounds, and careful judgment is needed in each case if one is to adopt a reasonable plan.

Although it is unusual in these cases for radiography to demonstrate a radiopaque foreign body, a patient with any puncture that penetrates through skin should also undergo radiographic examination at some time. Modern sophisticated techniques will on occasion reveal a small foreign body which entered at the time of puncturing. It is unfortunate to resort to surgical exploration belatedly only after continuing drainage has drawn attention to the probability of a retained foreign body, when that object would have been detectable on an initial radiograph. Although indications of bone or joint infection will not be evident initially, any superficial damage to bone produced by the nail itself may be demonstrated.

For every nail puncture wound seen in the hospital, many are sustained that are never seen medically. These are the most minor and superficial wounds, which heal readily and rapidly. For these clearly very minor injuries, aggressive warm soaks of the foot for a day or two will almost always suffice.

When there has been penetration through skin but probably not much deeper, vigorous soaking is warranted as well as careful observation to detect any developing inflammation.

If edema, tenderness, and redness develop around the puncture within a few hours, a 5- to 7-day, full-dosage course of an antibiotic or combination of antibiotics effective against *Staphylococcus aureus* and *Pseudomonas* is warranted, along with regular warm soaks. This is in the hope that there is cellulitis without foreign body retention. However, if there is not complete resolution of the reaction by the end of the course, exploration should be considered.

When a child is wearing running shoes at the time of the injury, there is a significant risk that a crumb of rubber from the sole of the shoe has been carried into the foot by the nail. A deep puncture caused by a nail passing through the sole of a running shoe, along with the onset of inflammation within a few hours, would be considered by many surgeons as good indication for primary exploration under antibiotic cover.

When exploration, either primary or at a later stage, is carried out, it can be done under local or general anesthesia, although one is wise to avoid local infiltration techniques if the inflammatory reaction is marked. The procedure will usually consist of excision of the cutaneous wound of entry, careful examination of the route through the underlying tissues if it can be visualized, meticulous search for and removal of any foreign material, the insertion of a satisfactory drain or packing, and dressing of the wound without suture closure. This should be done with the child in the prone position to provide access to the wound, and if general anesthesia has been selected, a tourniquet should be used to facilitate examination of the wound tract.

Although a finite course of antibiotic can be justified in an early infection, provided that the wound is carefully observed, one should not assume that antibiotic therapy is going to be the total answer. Potentially, every nail puncture wound is foreign body disease, and the risk of retention of foreign material makes it necessary to keep the need for exploration in mind at all times. For this reason, all puncture wounds other than the most minor merit an early surgical option, and subsequent treatment should be based on joint decisions.

Persistent drainage from a puncture wound after the inflammation has subsided, whether antibiotic has or has not been used, warrants exploration for retained foreign body.

A complication of nail puncture wounds that has been reported more frequently over the last few years is pseudomonas osteomyelitis, or septic arthritis. Factors which increase the incidence of this complication are location of the puncture over the metatarsal heads or distally and the passage of the nail through a running shoe sole before entering the foot.

The Spine

Cervical Fractures

General Considerations

Neck fractures are much less common in infants and young children than they are in adults. This may be partly due to greater mobility of the young neck but is probably also due to the relatively larger head and its greater tendency to be in the way, where it takes more of the brunt of the trauma.

Very rarely birth trauma has been known to cause a cervical fracture with quadriplegia. It is difficult to conceive of a more disabling injury. In general, it is remarkable what magnitude of stress can be sustained by the neonate's cervical spine during the delivery process without detectable damage.

Although teenagers sustain serious cervical cord damage in diving incidents or motorcycle accidents, these are quite comparable to those sustained by young adults and are not discussed further here.

On-Site Management

In any age group, suspicion of a cervical injury requires collar immobilization on site. Such suspicion is warranted if there is neck pain, anesthesia, paresthesia or weakness of an extremity, or a history suggestive of forces known to cause neck injuries, such as diving or a fall from a tree that results in landing on head and shoulder. A variety of sizes of collars for the pediatric age group are available and should be stocked on any prehospital vehicle. During transportation, the head should be strapped to the backboard as well because immobilization by collar is imperfect.

When prehospital care for head injuries is taught, care for the cervical spine is emphasized because of the risk of an associated unstable cervical fracture. For this reason, modified procedures, one of which is the nasotracheal route for intubation, are adopted in the control of airway out of respect for the neck. In infants and young children, not only is it recognized that head injuries are rarely accompanied by significant neck injuries, but also it is well known that airway maintenance can be very difficult in the small child. Consequently prehospital workers must assign top priority to the maintenance of airway and ventilation in children with head injuries, even if this results in more movement of the neck than one would be willing to accept in an adult. Airway and ventilation are critical in children, and in the absence of any evidence of a cervical injury one must never compromise respiration because of the fear that there might be an unsuspected cervical fracture associated with the head injury.

In adults who are comatose because of head trauma, blind nasotracheal intubation is frequently recommended to establish a secure airway while protecting the neck at the same time. This is not recommended for the young child or infant because of the amount of adenoidal tissue carried in by this procedure. In addition, nasal intubation in infancy requires a degree of skill rarely found at the accident site. Therefore, careful orotracheal intubation with the head held firmly in the "sniff" position is recommended for primary airway establishment in infancy and early childhood.

Primary Care

Many children who have sustained head injuries arrive in the hospital wearing cervical collars when there has been no suggestion of a neck injury. In others, some indication of neck injury is noted but only after the collar has been removed and the neck examined. Still others clearly require a full radiographic assessment before the collar is manipulated in any way.

In the instance in which a collar has been applied for no reason other than that the child was knocked down, provided that there is no cervical discomfort and no indication of nerve pressure or damage, the collar should be gently removed, the neck palpated for tenderness and deformity, and gentle movements permitted to assess pain on movement. The absence of any objective findings or complaints referable to the neck is justification for deferring any cervical radiographs at least for the present. If subsequent findings are noted, the collar should be reapplied and a good-quality lateral radiograph of the neck taken through the collar should be obtained before anything else is done.

If there is reason to suspect a neck injury, the lateral neck radiograph through the collar is just the first step. Only when it is pronounced normal by a clinician skilled in interpreting cervical radiographs may the collar be very gingerly removed and other appropriate views obtained. Flexion-extension lateral films may be necessary to demonstrate mild degrees of anterior instability. However, these views must be done with careful medical supervision and should be ordered only by the consulting service.

Definitive Therapy

In the presence of any neurologic symptoms or radiographic evidence of a cervical fracture, the child should be referred immediately to the appropriate surgical consultant, orthopaedist or neurosurgeon. Cervical immobilization must be maintained while the referral is being arranged.

Thoracolumbar Spinal Injuries

General Considerations

Injuries of any type to the thoracic or lumbar spine are unusual in pediatric practice, and cases with serious consequences are rare. In infancy or early childhood, spinal neurologic deficit is much more likely to be due to a congenital lesion involving the neural canal and its contents. Paraplegia or paraparesis due to a tumor of the cord or its coverings, or as a result of the surgical treatment of the tumor, is also encountered almost as frequently in a pediatric institution as is traumatic paraplegia.

As a result of the relative rarity of spinal trauma in pediatric practice, most cases which are encountered are referred early on to specialized centers, where greater experience has been accumulated. As a matter of fact, most major spinal trauma in the pediatric age group is encountered in the teenager, who has reached full stature and whose management is quite comparable to that provided for adults.

Thoracic or Lumbar Spinal Fractures

In the pediatric institution, fracture-dislocations of the thoracic or the lumbar spine causing major neurologic deficit are seen in the teenager from the same mechanisms of injury as are encountered in adult practice. Motorcycle accidents, collisions between motor vehicles and pedestrians, and those involving all-terrain vehicles are prime examples.

Prehospital management includes maintenance of in-line traction, secure immobilization by strapping to a backboard, and early transfer to a unit capable of handling major spinal trauma.

Initial medical assessment will include a careful search for other injuries and such intravenous fluid administration as is required for basic resuscitation. An indwelling urinary catheter on straight drainage will be needed both for management of shock and for decompression of the paralyzed bladder.

Continuing management, decisions regarding the need for surgical decompression or fusion at the fracture site, the sophisticated nursing care necessary for maintenance of skin health, and urinary management and related considerations are best handled in a spinal injury center. In such a center, ultimate rehabilitation to the optimum level possible is best obtained.

Compression Fractures

Compression fractures of one or of two adjacent vertebrae are common. This injury usually involves the middle to lower thoracic vertebrae or much less often the upper one or two lumbar vertebrae. Landing from a fall in the upright position, either standing or sitting, and being boarded in a hockey game in such a way as to produce a violent flexion stress are the common types of mechanisms of injury. The older child or teenager with a compression fracture of the thoracic spine may be able to walk into the department but will complain of pain over the injured spinal level and particularly pain on movement and deep breathing. There is not likely to be much of significance to find on examination except for a back which is held rigidly and pain on percussion over the site. The individual will be unwilling to flex the spine. Neurologic findings on examination and any neurologic sequelae are exceedingly rare.

Treatment consists of bed rest for the few days required for symptoms to resolve, followed by gradual resumption of full activity over the subsequent 4 to 6 weeks.

Spondylolysis and Spondylolisthesis

The defect in the pars interarticularis of L5 is characteristic of spondylolysis; L4 is involved in about 15 percent of instances. The defect, which is best visualized on the oblique radiographic projection as a "collar" or a "beheading" of a Scottish terrier, was long considered to be congenital. However, current thinking suggests the defects are acquired and likely the result of the recurrent trauma of weight bearing over a long time. Although sometimes blamed for chronic low back pain, it is unlikely that spondylolysis alone has significant clinical manifestations.

When the presence of a defect in the pars interarticularis bilaterally permits the body of L5, along with the pedicles and the superior articular facets, to shift forward on the sacrum, the condition termed "spondylolisthesis" is said to be present. Various degrees of slippage can occur, although a major shift is rare.

When a teenager, particularly female, is being examined radiographically for chronic pain at the lumbosacral level, the lateral film must be viewed with care to avoid missing even small degrees of forward slippage of L5. Oblique films to demonstrate spondylolysis should be considered.

The clinical significance of spondylolysis itself, or of small amounts of subsequent spondylolisthesis, is sufficiently controversial that orthopaedic referral is warranted for teenagers manifesting it. Spinal fusion to stabilize the L5 to S1 segment is rarely indicated.

Extradural Hematoma of the Spine

Extradural spinal hematomas are rare complications of what are usually totally innocuous injuries to the vertebrae, such as compression fractures of the lower thoracic vertebrae. When a dural vein is perforated during a lumbar puncture, an extradural collection of blood is always a possibility, although the risk is very small and almost exclusively restricted to the child with a bleeding diathesis. Whenever a known "bleeder" presents with a clinical picture that suggests meningitis, no lumbar puncture is permissible until the bleeding tendency has been corrected by administration of the appropriate factor and confirmation of its correction by the appropriate laboratory test. Some physicians would probably choose not to run even the small risk of a hematoma and would not include a lumbar puncture as part of the work-up on a child known to have a bleeding tendency of any sort.

Nontraumatic Spinal Conditions

General Considerations

Fewer children come to the emergency department because of acute back pain than is the case with adults, but when they do, the problem is almost always due to organic disease of the back, not a functional or psychosomatic condition. Furthermore, degenerative disk disease is rarely seen in children, although teenagers occasionally manifest it. Other causes of spondylogenic back pain, i.e., back pain originating in the spinal structures themselves, although well documented and described, are also relatively uncommon.

Viscerogenic back pain, or pain which is felt in the back but is caused by an intrathoracic or intra-abdominal lesion, such as aortic dissection, biliary colic, duodenal ulcer penetration, or pancreatic carcinoma, is almost exclusively a symptom of adulthood. Of the well-known visceral lesions causing pain in the back, biliary colic is almost the only example that does occasionally occur in the pediatric age group, although even it is virtually restricted to the teenage years. Rarely must one look further than the spine itself when seeking the cause of back pain in children.

Although examination of the back is not routinely necessary in a pediatric emergency department, spinal posture sometimes does provide a clue to the diagnosis of an underlying condition, and it behooves the emergency physician to be aware of the several possibilities. Marked lordosis or hyperextension of the lumbar spine may be evidence of a flexion contracture of the hip because the pelvis rotates forward in the attempt to mask the hip flexion. Lordosis may also be a manifestation of the spinal muscular weakness of a neurologic disorder such as muscular dystrophy.

Lumbar Disk Herniation

Herniation of a lumbar intervertebral disk, with full-blown sciatic pain and evidence of root tension and pressure, is occasionally seen in the teenager, although much less often than in the adult. There have probably been many teenagers with back pain due to undiagnosed disk disease who should be more easily identified now with the availability of more sophisticated imaging techniques. Fortunately the basic lesion is almost always a bulge only, not a fragment sequestration, and there is usually excellent response to several weeks of bed rest.

Spinal Osteitis

The term "spinal osteitis" usually refers to a characteristic form of staphylococcal osteomyelitis of vertebral bodies seen particularly in the young child. Presumably of hematogenous origin, this condition occurs with back pain, a rigid thoracolumbar spine, and some pain with vigorous percussion of the lower thoracic and upper lumbar spine but only mild systemic signs of infection. The sedimentation rate is usually moderately to markedly elevated.

This is an uncommon condition, and punch biopsy of the affected vertebral body is usually required to establish the diagnosis. Complete recovery is generally obtained with aggressive parenteral antibiotic therapy. This lesion generally does not suppurate, and surgical drainage is rarely necessary.

Adolescent Kyphosis
(Scheuermann's Disease)

Adolescent kyphosis, or Scheuermann's disease, is a fairly common chronic condition that can, on occasion, produce back pain leading to an emergency department visit. In this disease, there is growth disturbance of the anterior portions of both the upper and the lower epiphyseal plates of each affected vertebral body. Because these are the epiphyses that provide for growth in height, this disturbance causes slowing of the anterior growth and, consequently, gradually increasing kyphosis. A compensatory increased lumbar lordosis is often noted as well.

Scheuermann's disease most often affects several adjacent vertebrae in the lower thoracic and upper lumbar regions. It generally begins in the early teens and continues until growth has finished. Although the active process subsides completely at the time of epiphyseal fusion, the degree of deformity that has developed persists. Hence, early orthopaedic advice and management are important in the hope of minimizing deformity.

Myelomeningocele

Newborns with meningoceles or other variants of the spina bifida group of anomalies rarely appear primarily in the emergency department. They are usually seen in the neonatal unit and referred directly for surgery. When such a child is seen in the emergency department, the reason for the visit is likely to be a complication of the basic neural tube defect. These conditions fall into two main categories: myelomeningocele related to paraplegia and myelomeningocele related to hydrocephalus.

Myelomeningocele Related to Paraplegia

As a result of disuse osteomalacia, long bone fractures are relatively common in children who are congenitally paraplegic because of myelomeningoceles. Although the femur is most commonly broken, fractured tibias are also seen. Because of the lack of normal sensory perception, these injuries may be present for several days before medical help is sought. The first indication to the parent that something is amiss may be the observation of a hard mass in the thigh. These fractures usually heal uneventfully. If the child does not bear weight on the legs, a degree of deformity can be accepted that would otherwise require reduction. A form of treatment is usually selected that returns the child to a normal level of activity as soon as possible.

Pressure sores can occur but are much less common than is the case with paraplegia in adulthood.

Because of residual urine and frequent need for intermittent catheterization, urinary tract infections are very common in these children. As a result, any paraplegic, febrile child with no apparent cause for the fever should be assumed to have a urinary infection until samples can be obtained to prove or disprove it.

Myelomeningocele Related to Hydrocephalus

Most children born with myelomeningoceles also have the Arnold-Chiari malformation, in which the cerebellar tonsils protrude down through the foramen magnum beside the medulla. This is usually associated with an obstructive hydrocephalus that manifests any time in the first few months of life and usually requires surgical decompression by way of a shunt beginning in a cerebral ventricle which runs subcutaneously to either the abdomen or the right atrium.

Consequently several weeks or months after a meningocele has been surgically repaired, an emergency physician might see a young baby who is showing the early signs of hydrocephalus, with enlarging head and spread sutures. Alternatively, and much more commonly, will be the child who has been treated surgically but whose shunt is malfunctioning, either from breakage of the tube itself or from plugging of the lumen at the cerebral or distal end. Gentle manipulation of the subcutaneous pump-valve as it lies under the scalp will usually indicate whether there is a lag in filling or resistance to outflow, thus identifying obstruction at upper or lower ends, respectively.

Respiratory arrest episodes are also described in children with myelomeningoceles because of the intermittent tendency for the medulla and the cerebellar tonsils to plug the foramen magnum, resulting in temporary pressure on the medulla and depression of the respiratory control center. This causes sudden and unexpected cessation of respirations, lasting a few minutes, in a child who had a myelomeningocele operated on in infancy but who may or may not have had clinical hydrocephalus. The emergency physician should be aware of this complication so that if such a child is resuscitated in the department, neurosurgical referral can be instituted to permit consideration of surgical exposure and enlargement of the foramen.

Midline Dermal Sinus

Ideally midline dermal sinuses are discovered at routine neonatal examination. However, some are so inconspicuous as not to be seen, or their significance is not known. The midline dermal sinus runs deeply from the skin surface, in the midline, for a variable distance. Characteristically, however, it extends right into the subarachnoid space and therefore provides potential bacterial access to the spinal canal. In the absence of an underlying immunologic defect, a midline dermal sinus would be a likely cause of recurrent meningitis in the baby or young child. Although most such dermal sinuses are in the lumbar area, they can occur anywhere throughout the length of the spine and are reported from time to time over the skull or face but always in the midline.

The cutaneous end of a midline dermal sinus can usually be recognized from the tiny visible punctum that is the opening itself, a tuft of hair protruding from it, or a small pigmented spot. When such a sinus is noted, urgent neurosurgical referral is warranted because total excision of the sinus becomes much more difficult after it has been infected.

Diastematomyelia

When a 2- or 3-year-old child presents with a gait disturbance of recent onset that is worsening as well as spasticity and other long tract signs, the diagnosis of diastematomyelia should be considered. In this congenital condition, a spicule of bone traverses the neural canal in the anteroposterior direction, transfixing the cord and tethering it at that level. When the longitudinal growth spurt occurs in the 2- or 3-year-old, traction is put on the cord with the resultant long tract signs. Although recently introduced radiographic techniques are much

more effective at demonstrating this lesion than were the conventional methods, recognizing that there is a neurologic deficit underlying
the gait disturbance is of the greatest importance and is the single most
important step in the ladder to neurosurgical treatment.

Other Causes of Progressive Spinal Neurologic Disability

Diastematomyelia might be considered a prototype of a number of conditions of the lower spinal cord that can result in gait disturbances,
bowel or bladder dysfunction, ascending paraparesis, and paraplegia.
These conditions necessitate detailed radiographic techniques and
probably laminectomy before definitive diagnosis can be reached.
Some of the possibilities are hemangioma or arteriovenous malformation, spinal cord tumor, or an extradural tumor such as a "collar-
button" neuroblastoma with a small intraspinal extension of the much
larger intra-abdominal mass.

The spinal extradural hematoma typically occurs in this manner
as well, although its course is usually a matter of hours and not days.
Although rare, extradural hematomas are so amenable to surgical
decompression if treated in time that awareness of the condition is essential. For example, one must be alert to the possibility of an extradural hematoma in a child who develops progressive signs a few
hours after sustaining a vertebral compression fracture.

When the lumbar puncture needle tears an extradural vessel, the
resultant bleeding can theoretically produce a clot, which compresses the cord. Fortunately this is extremely rare in the child who is otherwise normal. However, lumbar puncture in a child with hemophilia
or some other bleeding diathesis is known on occasion to result in
ascending paraplegia due to an expanding extradural hematoma. The
child with a bleeding or clotting defect should not have a lumbar puncture unless and until the defect is first corrected.

General Disorders

Multiple Injuries

In spite of increasing efforts directed at accident prevention, the establishment of special pediatric trauma centers, and growing awareness of the specific treatment needs of the injured child, trauma continues to outnumber all other causes of death in the pediatric population.

As a result of the belated recognition of this "epidemic," most Advanced Trauma Life Support (ATLS) courses, which initially were directed exclusively at the adult patient population, now include pediatric modules, developed by and in most centers delivered by specialists experienced in pediatric trauma. This evolved, albeit somewhat belatedly, not only because of the inappropriateness of some of the routine procedures advised for adults when applied to the young child, but also because of increasing awareness of the sometimes unique ways in which accidents are caused in children and how the clinical manifestations of trauma in children differ from those seen in adults. Although still in its infancy, pediatric ATLS teaching is beginning to have benefit, and in more and more centers management designed for and appropriate to the child is being provided.

Causes

Although passenger restraint systems have been made compulsory in many jurisdictions and have decreased the incidence of injury caused by ejection, passenger deaths continue to outnumber pedestrian deaths in this jurisdiction. Ejection injuries can be expected to be the most serious of all vehicular accident injuries. A disturbing number of children of all ages are still severely traumatized as pedestrians when struck by moving vehicles. Young bicyclists are also frequent victims on city streets. The serious head injuries which so commonly occur in this way have prompted current recommendations regarding the wearing of protective helmets when cycling.

Nonvehicular urban accidents resulting in significant injury occur in many ways. Falls from balconies or windows on upper floors of apartments or from trees characteristically cause femoral fractures and internal damage in the abdomen or the chest. Small children frequently fall down long flights of stairs, not infrequently because of the extra mobility provided by a walker, and sustain damage to the skull and its contents.

Although in the rural population injuries due to vehicular accidents are still disturbingly common, serious injuries are also inflicted by farm machinery such as combines, grain augers, and tractors as well as lumbering equipment and road construction machinery. These "weapons" produce an unpredictable variety of lesions.

Child abuse must be kept in mind whenever a child is encountered whose injuries are not clearly and readily explained on the basis of a simple straightforward accident history. Life-threatening nonaccidental trauma is characteristically seen in the young baby in a home where the caregivers are young, inexperienced, and under great stress. All health care professionals must remain alert to the possibility of abuse if significant instances of child-battering are to be detected and adequate protection is to be offered.

Injury Patterns in the Multiple Injury Complex

In general, head injuries predominate in pediatric trauma and are associated with cervical fractures less often than in adult practice. Children injured by falling from heights or through contact with farm or other large machinery demonstrate injuries which are of such a variety of type and location that consistent patterns are very difficult to identify, if such patterns are present at all. However, for injured children who are struck as pedestrians by moving vehicles, there is an observed injury pattern resulting from the typical energy distribution inflicted by the moving vehicle. A general knowledge of this pattern can be of assistance in the early assessment of the injured child.

Over half of the children who sustain injuries when struck by a moving vehicle receive the energy of impact up one side of the body. A much smaller group of such children sustain injuries that either are distributed over both sides of the body or suggest that the trauma was sustained over the lower or upper half of the body without any particular lateralization.

It is also of interest that in those North American children whose injuries clearly demonstrate a unilateral distribution, the left side is involved twice as commonly as is the right. This is attributed to the fact that vehicles in the first lane of traffic entered when a child runs onto a roadway approach from the left. Although good statistical studies on this topic are lacking, physicians in Great Britain have indicated that the predominantly injured side there is the right, as would be expected from the side of the road on which vehicles are driven in Great Britain.

In attempts to ensure survival from major trauma in the pediatric age group, accurate diagnosis and prompt management of injuries sustained by intrathoracic or intra-abdominal viscera are of particular importance. With this in mind, attention to injury patterns has demonstrated that in the child showing apparent injuries up one side of the body the internal organ(s) likely to be injured is almost always on the same side as the visible external manifestations. This means that the child with an apparent femoral fracture on the left side and tire marks on the left lower chest is at high risk for both splenic injury and left traumatic pneumothorax. Similarly the child with a diagnosed right pneumothorax and right fractured femur following trauma should be repeatedly checked for an injury to the liver or the right kidney.

History

A brief history is very useful and is of greatest value when obtained prior to examination of the child. However, a detailed history of the mechanism of injury is often not obtainable until some time after the patient's arrival. If this is the case, a member of the treatment team should be released to take a history when an informant does arrive. As well as details concerning the accident itself, it is important to elicit information regarding past health, underlying disease, immunizations, allergies, and currently used medications.

Knowledge of the mechanism of the accident frequently suggests the most likely injuries and can alert one to a possible serious lesion, which could result in disastrous consequences if not anticipated and handled accordingly. The prime example of this is the cervical spine fracture sustained when the subject dives into too shallow water. In this situation, proper cervical immobilization will help to ensure against further cord damage with its neurologic sequelae and may even prevent cord damage if none has yet occurred.

The timing of an accident provides useful information regarding the rapidity of hemorrhage and onset of shock. An interval of 6 to 8 hours since the accident with still no indication of hypovolemia is strong evidence against hemorrhage of an alarming degree. This cannot be assumed if the seemingly normovolemic patient is seen within minutes of the incident.

Initial Assessment

One must approach the seriously injured child with a disciplined mind. It is necessary to ignore the obvious and dramatic but nonlife-threatening injuries, such as femoral fracture, facial laceration, and degloving injury to the arm. The assessment must be done in a priority sequence, first addressing physiologic derangements that can result in immediate or early death.

While evaluating the child initially, one must rely to the greatest extent on inspection to provide the critical information. The smaller the patient is, the more productive inspection becomes, relative to other modalities. Adult hands hide large areas of a small child's body from vision if applied too soon. One must not forget to stand back and look. Furthermore, while looking one should listen for abnormal respiratory noises as well as look for the abnormal respiratory movements.

If all is well, it is usually a simple matter to establish this fact, by looking for the most part, along with a little palpating and auscultating and some preliminary basic investigations. The following section describes the sequence that the assessment should follow.

Priority Sequence

With the possible exception of vigorous external hemorrhage or a visible open wound of the chest wall, both of which will in most instances be controlled by the receiving nurse before the physician arrives, there is nothing which should be permitted to command attention before the following essential sequence of vital matters is dealt with.

Airway

In most instances, looking and listening will provide the necessary information about airway patency. The gurgle or rattle of partial obstruction is usually obvious, as is total lack of any respiratory movement or sound. Vigorous inspiratory effort that serves only to suck the abdomen in, followed by attempted expiration that blows the abdomen out, with chest movements that are the opposite, suggests complete or near complete obstruction. One must remember that the lack of audible obstructive sounds is sometimes due to inadequate air exchange. If one wonders whether the ventilation is adequate, it probably is not.

The child who is deeply stuporous, or comatose, as a result of cerebral trauma (Glasgow Coma Scale of less than 7 or 8) requires early establishment of an artificial airway, preferably endotracheal. This protects the airway, which is in serious jeopardy in the semiconscious or unconscious individual, and provides a route not only for oxygen administration, but also for hyperventilation, which is important in counteracting the cerebral edema of hypoxia and hypercarbia. Establishment of an artificial airway also isolates the trachea from the esophagus lest regurgitation occur and lead to aspiration of vomitus.

Blind nasotracheal intubation is customary in adults because it permits intubation with less cervical manipulation than orotracheal intubation done under direct visualization of the glottis. In potential trauma to the neck, this is clearly safer. However, in the child under

10 or 12 years of age, the amount of soft adenoidal tissue in the pharynx is a deterrent to nasotracheal intubation. In addition, the glottis is more anterior and superior in the child and less accessible to blind nasal intubation. For this reason, gentle head manipulation into the "sniff" position followed by orotracheal intubation in the usual manner is recommended. The unexpected unstable cervical fracture in association with a head injury is uncommon in the pediatric age group, and one must not permit airway and ventilation to be compromised out of fear that obtaining an adequate airway will put at risk an as yet unsuspected cervical fracture.

Although the simple oropharyngeal airway easily overcomes pharyngeal obstruction caused by the tongue, it causes more airway resistance than the endotracheal tube. In addition, the oropharyngeal airway does not protect the trachea from regurgitated stomach contents. In the child whose level of consciousness is rising, the insertion of the oropharyngeal airway may induce regurgitation.

Head positioning and the use of the semiprone posture are time-honored techniques to maintain patency of the oropharyngeal air passages and provide a route for regurgitated matter to flow from the mouth. Although in many instances careful head positioning has been observed to maintain the airway fairly well during transportation, even over long distances, very close supervision is necessary. There is no provision for ventilation, and there is always very significant danger of aspiration. Particularly in adults, one would also be concerned that the required manipulations might jeopardize the cervical spine.

For these reasons, endotracheal intubation is indicated whenever transportation is required for a patient with depressed consciousness, even if drug-induced muscular relaxation is required for the intubation. This point is crucial and one cannot exaggerate its importance. Too often a physician accustomed to intubating unconscious adults is reluctant to intubate a comparably injured child, claiming that the child's breathing "seems okay to me." The most common error in preparing a seriously injured child for transportation is general reluctance to intubate the child in circumstances that, in adult practice, would be clear and mandatory indications for endotracheal intubation.

Breathing

The administration of oxygen to anyone with a serious truncal or cranial injury should be automatic. The method of administration will depend on airway patency and the possible need for positive pressure insufflation.

Inspection and auscultation usually provide a fairly good evaluation of respiratory exchange. However, these are educated guesses at best, and unless respiratory excursions are full and free and airway totally uncompromised, assisted ventilation through an artificial airway must be considered, especially in the presence of craniocerebral trauma. Arterial oxygen tension readings become important at this stage to evaluate respiratory exchange, although the first steps in resuscitation must not await the arrival of oxygen tension results. Arterial sampling has generally been necessary to obtain arterial gas tensions, although when perfusion is adequate, noninvasive percutaneous oxymetry is generally satisfactory and as time passes will doubtless be more widely used.

In the presence of a head injury, it is of particular importance to ensure adequate ventilation. Intubation and hyperventilation are indicated in the acute stage of most moderate to severe head injuries as prevention and treatment for cerebral edema. The most critical component of the early management of head injuries, even more important than craniotomy, which is infrequently needed, is care of the airway and maintenance of ventilation. Patients still suffer irreparable damage, and some probably still die, because of airway and respiratory care that is not sufficiently early or sufficiently aggressive. One cannot overemphasize this segment of patient care.

When there is indication of closed thoracic trauma, the respiratory compromise due to intrathoracic organ damage, such as traumatic pneumothorax or hemopneumothorax, should be anticipated and quickly recognized. It is important to diagnose the traumatic pneumothorax early because progression of the air leak can lead to massive pulmonary collapse, mediastinal displacement, and shock. A tension pneumothorax is one of the few true emergencies ever encountered and requires immediate drainage. (See Chapter 26 for further information on recognition and management of closed chest trauma).

Circulation

Early recognition of inadequate peripheral perfusion and immediate institution of rapid venous replacement of lost blood are the basic requirements for diagnosing and treating shock following trauma. Cardiac monitoring and continual blood pressure determinations are important and must be initiated as soon as possible. Although various automatic pressure manometers are useful in following arterial pressures, serial readings obtained by an experienced nurse using a conventional sphygmomanometer are completely satisfactory.

The clinical features indicating inadequate peripheral perfusion, the routes and methods for blood volume replacement, the fluid types and volumes required, and the indication for acid-base management are all covered in Chapter 45.

It should be emphasized that the bolus technique of fluid replacement is of particular value in cases of multiple trauma. When perfusion has been restored by prompt venous infusion but the presence of a second actively bleeding lesion cannot be excluded, subsequent deterioration after initial restoration of calculated blood volume, with the infusion running at maintenance only, is a strong signal to the physician that there is further bleeding.

When active infusion for presumed traumatic shock in a child with thoracic trauma does not produce the expected improvement in circulation, pericardial tamponade must be considered. S-T elevation and

T-wave flattening or inversion on the electrocardiogram, a globular shape to the cardiac shadow on X-ray film, and increasing central venous pressure, shown either by manometry or by jugular venous distention, singly or in combination, are clear indications for substernal aspiration of the pericardial sac. With the needle inserted just to the left of the xyphoid process, angled up and back at 45 degrees, the removal of sometimes surprisingly little fluid can correct the situation. Repeated aspirations or thoracotomy may be necessary if tamponade is due to a small cardiac wound that continues to bleed. To monitor the risk of the needle impinging on the ventricle and inducing dangerous arrhythmias, the V lead of the electrocardiogram may be connected to the needle. When myocardium is contacted by the needle, S-T elevation is produced and the needle can be withdrawn a little.

Increasing Intracranial Pressure

For practical purposes, progressive increase in intracranial pressure is the only other condition that might require care on a true emergency basis. Although established diffuse cerebral edema resulting from trauma, whether or not aggravated by hypoxia, is often not amenable to therapy, hyperventilation may reverse the process if initiated sufficiently early. Keeping blood carbon dioxide levels down and maintaining high oxygen tensions can also keep deterioration to a minimum while an accident victim is being transferred to a specialty center.

In addition, the clinical picture of delayed increased intracranial pressure following trauma can be due to an expanding surface clot, which may be treatable by surgical decompression. For a discussion of the clinical manifestations, diagnosis, and management of this complication of cranial trauma, see Chapter 17.

Completing the Assessment

Only when one can be certain that airway and ventilation are satisfactory, that rapid flow venous infusions have been established and fluid resuscitation is under way, and that there is no indication of increasing intracranial pressure requiring urgent measures is it reasonable to proceed with the rest of the examination. The secondary survey is a comprehensive head-to-toe examination and includes inspection, palpation, and auscultation. It is designed to reveal those injuries which do not threaten life on an emergency basis but, because such injuries cause continuing blood loss, tissue damage, and pain, result in continuing deterioration and can then be lethal in hours if not reversed.

The spectrum of injuries sustained is limitless, although certain examples are more common in children than others and should be expected and sought particularly. For an account of the more frequently encountered injuries in the abdomen, chest, pelvis, and extremities, see Chapters 21, 26, 31, 39, and 40.

Investigation

The standard investigations listed in the trauma protocol and carried out for most victims of major trauma are a basic series of blood tests and radiographs that can then be augmented or partially eliminated depending on the nature of the accident and the expected injuries.

In addition to obtaining blood for cross-matching, routine blood work includes assessment of the hemoglobin, white cell count and differential, hematocrit, glucose, urea, electrolytes, and amylase. Arterial oxygen and carbon dioxide levels are important with head or chest injuries, although percutaneous oxymetry can serve for this purpose in many instances. Although the routine of doing all the tests according to protocol, whatever the state of the patient, does introduce consistency and ensures that all needed information is likely to be obtained, one should remain open to modifications according to individual requirements. The child with bilateral femoral fractures who has no respiratory compromise will in most instances not require an arterial gas analysis, nor is there strong indication for a serum amylase determination in the child admitted with several fractures but neither symptoms nor signs referable to the abdomen.

Radiographic evaluation is very important but must not replace or delay careful physical assessment and clinical judgment. The clinician must not await radiographic confirmation of a tension pneumothorax before relieving intrapleural pressure, nor do plain skull radiographs contribute very often to the decision to proceed to immediate craniotomy for an extradural hemorrhage. However, emergency radiography has for many years contributed enormously to the overall evaluation of the injured child and should be obtained as soon as resuscitative needs have been satisfied. The initial films requested are (1) cross-table lateral view of the neck exposing down to C7 and (2) supine anteroposterior view of the chest. As treatment needs permit, others in order of importance are (3) anteroposterior view of the abdomen and (4) pelvis, (5) anteroposterior and lateral views of the skull, and (6) extremity views as indicated by examination. All these films should be obtained in the resuscitation room and require either a portable machine or a ceiling-mounted X-ray tube designed for the specific purpose.

A further and absolutely mandatory requirement is a competent interpretation of the films as soon as possible. The effort and time involved in obtaining the films and the difficulties in monitoring and treating the patient while radiographs are obtained are worthwhile only if the information obtainable from the films is immediately available for clinical use. Too often the obscure cervical fracture, the small collection of pleural fluid, or the suggestion of a small traumatic diaphragmatic hernia is not recognized until the following day. Sometimes the physicians involved do not learn promptly of the radiographic abnormalities because they do not see the films immediately themselves or because effective communication with the radiologist is lacking. The logistical preparations for management of major trauma must include such mundane matters as communication between clinician and radiologist.

As much as plain radiography has contributed to patient evaluation and management of major trauma over the years, newer and revolutionary modalities have now come into the forefront of trauma care. Computed tomography (CT) permits us to visualize, in three dimensions and high resolution, almost any internal organ. It demonstrates small visceral lacerations or collections of blood which are otherwise unsuspected. It localizes and identifies small isolated areas of edema or hemorrhage in the brain and displays in detail the configuration of complicated fracture lines as they cross pelvic bones, vertebrae, or skull. The CT machine is not, as yet, routinely available in many emergency departments. However, were this the case, it could easily and quickly exclude extradural hematomas and other conditions the risk from which leads to a net hospital stay for many children of many days. Fewer days of in-hospital observation will be required and the savings will be commensurate when this modality has become a practical emergency department tool.

Magnetic resonance imaging (MRI) has capabilities comparable to CT and many more. However, MRI remains very much an elective modality, and there may never come the time when it is freely and routinely available for emergency department practice.

Ultrasonography also effectively demonstrates organ configuration and will reveal defects caused by trauma. Its main virtue is the lack of penetrating electromagnetic radiation.

In special situations, nuclear scans provide information that is difficult to obtain in other ways. The chief purpose of nuclear scans is to demonstrate the presence of a blood supply to the tissue or organ in question.

Nuclear medicine studies have been available in special centers for approximately 30 years, and CT scans have been available for 20 years. Widespread use of ultrasonography in trauma is relatively new. Magnetic resonance imaging is just being launched and so has not as yet proved its place in the management of trauma.

Although all the high-profile developments, particularly in the diagnostic imaging specialties, have become almost routine in some centers and have added a great deal in the process of evaluation of the trauma patient, it will be regrettable if all physician decision making is removed. Not every patient fits even the most general protocol. There will always be the child who requires some form of investigation that necessitates medical judgment to identify and request. Conversely, there are already many tests done because they are included in the protocol but prove to be totally unnecessary. It behooves the physician directors of trauma programs to resist complete automation, so to speak, of assessment and management policies. Some physician input must be retained, and the judgment of the physician, particularly those with long experience, must be able to override the routines dictated by protocol when it is appropriate to do so. Only then will all patients receive care which is best for them in a fiscally responsible way.

Management Organization:
Trauma Team

The most important development in the management of major trauma has been the recognition of the need for and the designation of specially staffed and prepared trauma centers. The principles of care for head injuries, chest injuries, and abdominal injuries have not changed. What has changed is an emphasis on their management in an organized, integrated manner.

The main asset of a trauma center is the trauma team. This is the treatment team and consists of a specifically designated group of physicians, nurses, and technicians representing the chief medical divisions and departments involved in the care of the seriously injured victim.

In the adult hospital, the physician component of the team usually consists of the trauma team leader, who is frequently a general surgeon, the emergency physician, and representatives from the most frequently involved surgical specialties, such as orthopaedics and general surgery. Other specialties, such as neurosurgery and plastic surgery, may be represented on the team or may remain available for calls from the team. The less frequently needed surgical specialties must also be available for the designation of trauma center to apply. Anesthetic specialists or intensivists are also very important and provide the highly skilled airway and ventilatory care so crucial to victims of serious trauma. The trauma protocol also provides for immediately available consultation services from the radiology department as well as the hematology department and the blood bank. Finally, in the interests of the victim's close family, trauma care cannot be considered complete without prompt assistance from social service or the chaplaincy service. In most trauma centers, a social worker or the on-call chaplain is called along with the other members of the trauma team.

In the pediatric institution, the basic makeup of the trauma team is similar to that in the adult center. In addition, however, general pediatrics has a major contribution to offer, mainly in the areas of general care for underlying illness, nutritional concerns, and, especially with the young child, expertise in obtaining rapid venous access. Where the pediatric input is provided by those specializing in emergency care, however, much more can be provided by the pediatrician, including major contributions in the areas of initial assessment and resuscitation. Specific assignment of responsibilities varies from hospital to hospital.

During a trauma resuscitation each member has specific duties to be carried out, all under the supervision of the trauma team leader. Some systems direct one individual to a specific side of the patient and give him or her two or three specific parameters to monitor and several specific technical procedures to perform. The team leader remains responsible for overall direction, judgment decisions, and treatment orders. In other systems, a more flexible approach is adopted, and much is left to the trauma team leader to delegate on the scene.

The only other general step toward better trauma care of an importance comparable to the establishment of trauma centers has been the development of specific courses in the initial management of trauma victims: the ATLS courses. These have proved to be particularly valuable for physicians working in smaller hospitals, where immediate backup from all the appropriate specialists is rarely available. Pediatric modules in the ATLS courses have also now been developed in the hope of providing for the young trauma victim the same quality of initial care that is available for adults under the ATLS teaching. Anyone who might be responsible for the reception and initial care of seriously injured patients, adult or child, is well advised to take an ATLS course and to be prepared to use the principles embodied in its teaching.

Parents

In emergency pediatric practice, the child is usually accompanied by one or both parents, who can give history and provide some support for the child as well as needed supervision when the physician or nurse is out of the room. However, when a child is received who has been seriously injured, he or she usually comes by ambulance and may be followed by parents to the hospital. Alternatively efforts may be required after the child's arrival to contact parents and inform them of the accident. Whatever the case, parents often have been separated from their child during transfer to the referral center or perhaps have not even seen the child since the accident.

For these reasons and because the term "serious injuries" always connotes to parents the possibility of fatality, special efforts are mandatory not only to be sensitive and gentle when obtaining relevant medical history from them, but also to keep them informed with as much support, kindness, and comfort as can be mustered. When a child is seriously injured, the doubts about the future initiate the early stages of the grieving process usually associated with the death of a loved one. Denial, anger, and questioning are all seen and must be received with understanding. Even when children survive potentially serious accidents unharmed, one must assume that the doubts and fears in the hearts of parents as they await the outcome are a stress of a severity rarely matched by anything short of bereavement.

A "quiet room" where family members can be interviewed in private is essential. It should be adjacent to the treatment area but not in the "heat of the action." Here parents can also make telephone calls, compose themselves after receiving bad news, or display emotions in a way they might not consider appropriate in public.

An emotional support service for distraught or grieving parents, such as an experienced social worker or an appropriate member of the clergy, can be of immeasurable help. It is also helpful to the physician to know that the parents are being cared for when he or she must leave them to return to the child.

Reassurance to parents must be honest. One must not be falsely encouraging when the outcome does not justify it. It is better for a parent to expect the worst and be subsequently encouraged than to have false hopes which are later dashed.

It is generally not practicable for a parent to be in attendance during resuscitation or other complicated procedures. On the other hand, one should try to arrange for a parent to be with the child when circumstances permit. Most parents are able to summon the strength to be calm and supportive when with the child. Furthermore, it is reassuring for a parent to see the careful and repeated examinations so often needed in monitoring the seriously injured and, ideally, to observe the child improving in response to treatment measures.

Even when there is no hope, the grieving process proceeds in a more healthy manner if the parent has had the opportunity to see and touch the dying child or, with a baby or a toddler, even to hold the body.

Fortunately the outcome in many trauma resuscitations is excellent, and the physicians involved have the privilege of feeling one of medicine's greatest satisfactions, that of seeing a child live and go home as the result of one's efforts. Remember that seeing this happen is also the greatest thrill a parent can receive. Playing a part in a successful resuscitation makes them all worthwhile, even those that are not successful.

Hypovolemic Shock

Causes

Hypovolemic shock can result from dehydration of excessive diarrhea or vomiting or from intraperitoneal losses subsequent to intestinal perforation. However, shock that is relevant to a surgical presentation is virtually restricted to that caused by large area burns or major mechanical trauma.

The large area burn causes shock through massive leaking of fluid from small blood vessels into the interstitial space around them. That damaged capillaries within the burn area are rendered abnormally permeable has been long understood. What has been more recently recognized is that in the presence of a large area burn, small vessels throughout the body generally also become excessively permeable. This is felt to be one effect of a circulating humoral factor released in response to the burn. For further information, the reader is directed to Chapter 5.

The usual cause of hypovolemic shock is hemorrhage from injured tissue in which blood is released directly from ruptured blood vessels either to the exterior or into body spaces such as the abdominal cavity or the chest.

In adults, hemorrhage into the extremities, such as can be expected to occur around a fractured femur, can readily be in an amount sufficient to cause shock. It should be emphasized that this situation is most unusual in the child. Extremity injuries alone rarely cause shock in the child, unless a major extremity vessel, such as the femoral artery, has been lacerated and is actively bleeding to the outside. The reasons for this are unclear, although it is easy to speculate that the child's arterial vessels contract more effectively than those of the adult and release less blood into the soft tissues around a fracture. If the young child with a fractured femur begins to manifest the clinical signs and symptoms of hypovolemia, the physician should look carefully elsewhere for the injury causing the hemorrhage before attributing it to the extremity injury alone.

In children, the common injury sites which can bleed to a serious degree are liver, spleen, kidney, and lung. From time to time pelvic fractures also result in massive hemorrhage but not as frequently as is seen in adults.

Multiple lacerations rarely result in hypovolemic shock in the child, although scalp lacerations may be the exception. They occasionally bleed massively and require pressure dressings for initial control and sometimes transfusion before definitive repair can be carried out.

It should be emphasized that, as is the case with adults, *head injuries do not cause shock*. Only if the cerebral injury is so severe that the child is near death will it be at all likely for shock to be due to the head injury. In such instances one should assume hypovolemic shock to be due to hemorrhage into the abdomen or the chest.

Pericardial tamponade can produce a clinical picture difficult to differentiate from shock due to blood loss. This should be suspected whenever trauma to the chest results in hypotension in the absence of adequate evidence of active intrapleural or intrapulmonary hemorrhage.

Clinical Manifestations

The basic symptoms and signs of hypovolemic shock are common to all age groups. However, in children, to avoid delays in making the diagnosis of shock in the early stages, greater emphasis must be placed on certain features which in adults are of less importance.

Pallor and extremities that are cold and clammy are the early signs of acute blood loss in children and may precede the onset of tachycardia and hypotension for a significant period. A child may lose up to a quarter of normal circulating blood volume before he or she shows a recognizable change in pulse rate or blood pressure. Any child in the recumbent position who demonstrates definite pallor and increased sweating after trauma must be assumed to have lost up to a quarter of blood volume even though pulse and blood pressure seem unchanged. Hypotension and tachycardia on the assumption of the sitting position can also be interpreted to indicate a moderate blood loss, although this is not a useful test for the majority of traumatized patients.

When hypotension is evident, blood loss is usually greater than a quarter of blood volume, and compensatory mechanisms can be expected to fail soon unless measures to replace fluid and control hemorrhage can be initiated at once.

In the younger age group, hypovolemic shock often produces an unusual form of confusion and inappropriate behavior not generally seen in other situations. The child may complain bitterly of the venous infusion site or a small peripheral abrasion while ignoring a broken femur or the pain of a splenic rupture. Repeated attempts to remove the oxygen mask or dressings on minor wounds are sometimes noted in spite of continued efforts to explain everything to the child and seek cooperation. That this is a manifestation of cerebral hypoxia and not because the child is basically ill-behaved or uncooperative is evident when behavior becomes completely appropriate coincident with restoration of normal tissue perfusion. Air hunger is noted, as it is in adult practice, and thirst is also complained of from time to time.

Treatment

Although the definitive treatment measure for blood loss is blood replacement, there are a number of other measures that are also of importance and must not be neglected.

Oxygen by mask should be started within seconds of the diagnosis being made if the child is conscious and breathing spontaneously. If the child is unconscious and in need of respiratory support, this is of top priority. If the child is ventilated, it will be a simple matter to ensure a high flow of oxygen. In addition, shock cannot be satisfactorily treated if a chest injury continues to compromise gas exchange. Hence, drainage of a pneumothorax or a large pleural collection must be accomplished immediately. Arterial oxygen levels can be monitored by percutaneous oxymetry painlessly and more easily than by arterial needle samples. Thus, where it is available, percutaneous oxymetry has virtually replaced intermittent arterial sampling by needle.

External hemorrhage must be controlled promptly by pressure. Unfortunately most exsanguination hemorrhage is not to the exterior and is not available to external control.

Appropriate splinting of major fractures helps greatly to decrease pain and avoid further soft tissue damage and bleeding around the fractures. However, fractures must not receive attention before adequate gas exchange is ensured and fluid resuscitation is well under way.

The institution of at least one, if not several large-bore venous infusions must be coincident with airway care and with ventilatory support when it is required. When immediate venous access is unobtainable, intraosseous infusion, usually into the tibial marrow space, is an effective alternative.

A number of different fluids have been recommended for initial resuscitation purposes. However, for the hypovolemic child, a balanced saline solution, such as Ringer's lactate, followed by whole blood when it is available, is generally quite satisfactory.

Ideally, any blood administered should be fully cross-matched against the child's blood. However, the degree of urgency will dictate if it is reasonable to await full cross-matching; if a quick cross will be necessary, in which case blood can often be available within 15 or 20 minutes; or if uncrossed, universal donor blood (type O negative) must be administered at once. An important determining factor in this decision is one's ability to control further bleeding. When bleeding can be expected to continue until open operation permits its control, whole blood is essential and uncrossed type O negative blood will probably be needed until fully cross-matched blood is available. If the hemorrhage can be stanched by simple measures in the emergency department, early shock can probably be managed initially with electrolyte solution, and it is likely to be safe to defer the decision to give blood until fully crossed blood is available.

Infusion volumes depend on the size of the child and the estimated volume of blood lost. For early to moderate shock, infusion fluid should be given in boluses roughly equal to one-fourth of the normal blood volume. This works out to approximately 20 ml per kilogram of body weight. The initial bolus should be infused as rapidly as possible, after which the child should be assessed and the decision made as to further fluid. If more is needed, it should be given as a similar bolus or boluses.

When circulation has been returned to normal, the infusion should be slowed down to maintenance speed and the clinical picture monitored carefully. If bleeding is continuing, tissue perfusion will deteriorate again and the need for further measures will be apparent. Too often the infusion is ill-advisedly left running briskly after perfusion has been restored. Continued bleeding may not become apparent for a while, masked as it is by the continued rapid infusion.

Concern about the metabolic acidosis of shock has in the past prompted aggressive treatment with buffer solutions, usually bicarbonate. It is now believed that, unless it is very marked, the acidosis is more safely managed in many instances by active restoration of blood volume and normal perfusion, which should induce spontaneous correction of the acidosis by normal physiologic processes. Notwithstanding this, many in the field will give at least one dose (0.5 to 1 ml per kilogram of the 7.5 percent solution) of bicarbonate at the start of the resuscitation to begin the reversal of the pH depression. Some continue to advise repeating such doses at arbitrary intervals, such as each half hour, for the period that clinical shock remains evident.

Throughout resuscitation, care should be taken to avoid permitting the child's core temperature to drop significantly. Air-conditioned treatment rooms, exposure for adequate examination and treatment, infusion of cool liquids, and underperfusion of heat-producing organs all lead to hypothermia. Although controlled hypothermia is beneficial in some situations, children tolerate badly the accidental hypothermia encountered during resuscitation procedures, and active measures to prevent it are important. Continual monitoring of body temperature; heat lamps, especially for the small child; warming of blood and other infusates; and avoidance of unnecessary exposure of the child all serve to detect and prevent accidental cooling during therapeutic procedures.

Resuscitation of the child suffering from hypovolemic shock implies sophisticated care delivered by a closely working team. Unfortunately such teams are not always available, leaving the care to one or two individuals who may have varying degrees of experience and confidence in dealing with the seriously injured child. However, principles of resuscitation are common to all ages, and if the physician observes the known differences described previously between children and adults and their responses to trauma and the resuscitative maneuvers employed, the child will be well served. Furthermore, in most situations the physician in the primary hospital will have access by telephone to those experienced in pediatric resuscitation so that initial resuscitation can be implemented before the physician transfers the child to their care.

Suggested Reading

The following list includes selected texts, major review articles, monographs, and some original journal articles, all of which make significant contributions to the literature on pediatric emergency surgical care. This is not a comprehensive list but should provide a spectrum of opinion extensive enough for most readers. The reader will recognize points presented in some of the publications listed here with which this author disagrees or to which he applies a different priority. In most instances, opposing opinions are based on differing degrees of pediatric orientation.

Many texts or manuals on emergency surgery or emergency care in general are also available. However, because the reader is expected to come to this book with a general knowledge base, both practical and theoretical, in adult emergency practice, these are not listed.

Comprehensive References

Abelson and Smith, eds. Residents Handbook of Pediatrics. 7th ed. Toronto: BC Decker, 1987.

Black, ed. Paediatric Emergencies. 2nd ed. London: Butterworths, 1987.

Fleischer and Ludwig, eds. Textbook of Pediatric Emergency Medicine. 2nd ed. Baltimore: Williams & Wilkins, 1988.

Welch and Randolph, eds. Pediatric Surgery. Vols I and II. Chicago: Year Book, 1986.

Pediatric Radiology

Gwinn and Stanley. Diagnostic Imaging in Pediatric Trauma. New York: Springer, 1980.

Wounds, Including Burns

Carvajal and Parks. Burns in Children, Pediatric Burn Management. Chicago: Year Book, 1988.

Goldin. Plastic Surgery (Pocket Consultant). Cambridge, MA: Blackwell, 1987.

Grabb and Smith. Plastic Surgery. Boston: Little, Brown, 1979.

McKinney and Cunningham. Handbook of Plastic Surgery. Baltimore: Williams & Wilkins, 1981.

Moore, ed. Early Care of the Injured Patient. Philadelphia: BC Decker, 1990. Especially Edlich. Chapter 24. Wounds. Edlich. Chapter 25. Bites and stings. Pruitt and Goodwin. Chapter 26. Burn injury.

Zuker. Helping the burned child. Emerg Care 1986.

Zukin and Simon. Emergency Wound Care: Principles and Practice. Rockville, MD: Aspen, 1987.

Ocular Emergencies

Crawford and Morin, eds. The Eye in Childhood. New York: Grune & Stratton, 1983. Especially Pashby and Chisholm. Chapter 15. Trauma.

Harley, ed. Pediatric Ophthalmology. Vols. I and II. 2nd ed. Philadelphia: WB Saunders, 1983.

Helveston and Ellis. Pediatric Ophthalmology Practice. 2nd ed. St. Louis: CV Mosby, 1984.

Vinger, ed. Ocular Sports Injuries. Internat Ophthal Clin 1981; Vol 21.

Dental Emergencies

Andersson and Bodin. Avulsed human teeth replanted within fifteen minutes: A long-term clinical follow-up study. Endod Dent Traumatol 1990; 6:37.

Andreasen. Traumatic Injuries of the Teeth. 2nd ed. Copenhagen: Munksgaard, 1981.

Topazian and Goldberg. Management of Infections of the Oral and Maxillofacial Regions. Philadelphia: WB Saunders, 1981.

Head Injuries

Bruce, Raphaely, Goldberg, et al. The pathophysiology, treatment and outcome following severe head injury in children. Child's Brain 1979; 5:174.

Caffey. The whiplash-shaken infant syndrome: Manual shaking of the extremities with whiplash induced intracranial and intraocular bleeding, linked with residual brain damage and mental retardation. Pediatrics 1974; 54:396.

Choux, Grisoli, Peragut. Extradural hematomas in children. 104 Cases. Child's Brain 1975; 1:337.

Hendrick, Harwood-Nash, and Hudson. Head injuries in children: A survey of 4465 consecutive cases at the Hospital for Sick Children, Toronto, Canada. Clin Neurosurg 1964; 11:46.

Ito, Miwa, and Onodra. Growing skull fracture of childhood with reference to the importance of brain injury and its pathogenetic consideration. Child's Brain 1977; 3:116.

Shapiro, ed. Pediatric Head Trauma. Mt. Kisco, New York: Futura, 1983.

Abdominal Trauma

Mayer, ed. Emergency Management of Pediatric Trauma. Philadelphia: WB Saunders, 1985. Especially Matlak. Chapter 20. Abdominal injuries.

Wesson. Abdominal injuries in children. Can J Surg 1984; 27:472.

Thoracic Trauma

Burrington. Chest injuries in children. Can J Surg 1984; 27:466.

Mayer, ed. Emergency Management of Pediatric Trauma. Philadelphia: WB Saunders, 1985. Especially Jones. Chapter 15. Thoracic trauma.

Nakayama, Raminovsky, Rowe. Chest injuries in childhood. Ann Surg 1989; 210:770.

Gynecologic Emergencies

1988 Canadian Guidelines for the Treatment of Sexually Transmitted Diseases in Neonates, Children, Adolescents and Adults. Canadian Diseases Weekly Report 1988; 14(Suppl):s2.

Cowell. The gynecologic examination of infants, children, and young adolescents. Ped Clin North Am 1981; 28:247.

Edmonds. Dewhurst's Practical Paediatric and Adolescent Gynaecology. 2nd ed. London: Butterworths, 1989.

Herriot, Emans, and Goldstein. Pediatric and Adolescent Gynecology. 2nd ed. Boston: Little, Brown, 1982.

Extremity Trauma and Fractures

Rang. Children's Fractures. 2nd ed. Philadelphia: JB Lippincott, 1983.

Salter. Textbook of Disorders and Injuries of the Musculoskeletal System. 2nd ed. Baltimore: Williams & Wilkins, 1983.

General Aspects of Pediatric Trauma

Burtain, Lynch, and Ramenovsky. Trauma. Vol 2. Chicago: Year Book, 1987.

Harris, ed. Proceedings of the First National Conference on Pediatric Trauma. Ped Emerg Care 1986; 2:113.

Harris, Latchaw, Murphy, and Schwaitzberg. A protocol for pediatric trauma receiving units. J Ped Surg 1989; 24:419.

Mattox, Moore, and Feliciano, eds. Trauma. East Norwalk, CT: Appleton & Lange, 1988. Especially Hatter and Pokorny. Chapter 44. Pediatric trauma.

Moore, ed. Early Care of the Injured Patient. Philadelphia: BC Decker, 1990. Especially Ramenofsky. Chapter 28. Pediatric trauma.

Ruddy and Fleischer. Pediatric trauma: An approach to the injured child. Ped Emerg Care 1986; 2:151.

Hypovolemic Shock

Eichelberger and Pratsch, eds. Pediatric Trauma Care. Rockville, MD: Aspen, 1988. Especially Mangulat and Eichelberger. Chapter 7. Hypovolemic shock in the pediatric trauma patient: A physiologic approach to diagnoses and treatment.

Mayer, ed. Emergency Management of Pediatric Trauma. Philadelphia: WB Saunders, 1985. Especially Mayer. Chapter 2. Management of hypovolemic shock.